CORONARY HEART DISEASE

A GUIDE *to* DIAGNOSIS *and* TREATMENT

BARRY M. COHEN, M.D. • BOBBIE HASSELBRING

Addicus Books
Omaha, Nebraska

An Addicus Nonfiction Book

ISBN 1-886039-58-5
Cover design by George Foster
Illustrations by Jack Kusler

This book is not intended to serve as a substitute for a physician, nor do the authors intend to offer medical advice contrary to that of an attending physician.

Library of Congress Cataloging-in-Publication Data

Cohen, Barry M.
    Coronary heart disease : a guide to diagnosis and treatment / Barry M.
Cohen, Bobbie Hasselbring.
        p. cm.
Includes index.
    ISBN 1-886039-58-5
    1. Coronary heart disease—Popular works. I. Hasselbring, Bobbie,
1951- II. Title.
    RC685.C6 C58 2002
    616.1'23—dc21
        2001007104

Addicus Books, Inc.
P.O. Box 45327
Omaha, Nebraska 68145
Web site: http://www.AddicusBooks.com

Printed in the United States of America
10 9 8 7 6 5 4 3 2 1

To my wife Jill,
and our children—Sara, Brett, and Chloe—
for their love and support
—BC

To Anne, always,
and to Max, Scout, Greta, and Bib
—BH

Contents

Foreword

More people are affected by atherosclerosis, commonly referred to as "hardening of the arteries," than by any other single disorder. We hear about the effects of atherosclerosis on the nightly news—strokes, loss of limbs, heart attack, and deaths. Our friends and family tell stories about those who have been touched by or even killed by atherosclerosis. Though you may worry more about cancer, you should be more concerned about heart disease, stroke, and leg artery disease.

Atherosclerosis doesn't affect just the heart. It affects the entire body. If you have a blockage in one artery, odds are that you have blockages in other arteries elsewhere in the body. For instance, if you have leg artery blockage, there is a 50/50 chance that you also have heart artery blockage. If you have heart artery blockage, there is a 30 percent chance that you have significant blockage of the artery that brings blood to the brain.

This is what makes early diagnosis and aggressive prevention the key to surviving atherosclerosis and coronary heart disease (CHD). This book is designed to help you understand what a heart attack means, how doctors can help you figure out if you have heart artery blockage even if you don't have symptoms, and what treatments are available. *Coronary Heart Disease: A Guide to Diagnosis and Treatment* will help you understand why smoking is so bad for you and how lowering your high cholesterol is an excellent method of reducing your risk of heart attack and death from CHD.

This book—designed for you, the patient—gives you valuable and up-to-date information, your most powerful weapon against atherosclerosis and heart disease. I urge you to read every page—for your good health and for your heart's good health.

Michael R. Jaff, D.O.
President-Elect, Society
for Vascular Medicine and Biology

Acknowledgments

No book is the work of the authors alone. We'd like to thank several of Dr. Cohen's colleagues for their invaluable assistance and insights: Drs. Mark Blum, Harvey Hecht, James London, Roberto Roberti, Alejandro Rodriguez, John Banas, and Carl Hess. Additionally, Dr. Cohen is indebted to his former professors—Dr. Valentin Fuster and the faculty at the Mount Sinai Medical Center in New York, Drs. Maurice Buchbinder and L. Kirk Peterson at the University of California San Diego Medical Center, Drs. Harold Frank, Seymour Cohen, and Irwin Labin for their wisdom, expertise, and inspiration. Dr. Cohen is also deeply appreciative of his parents, Elaine and Gerry Cohen for their support and guidance.

The authors would also like to thank our publisher, Rod Colvin of Addicus Books, for his infinite patience, his fine editing skills, and his clear vision for the book. Without you, this project would not be a reality.

Most of all, we'd like to thank Dr. Cohen's many patients. It is you who have provided the experience, the insight, and the humanity that makes the work worthwhile.

Introduction

Coronary heart disease (CHD) is the number one killer in North America. Although there isn't a cure yet, there are many excellent treatments available to control symptoms and help people live long and healthy lives. We now have the technology to detect CHD early, even before you have symptoms, which may help decrease your risk of a heart attack. That is why we wrote this book—to give you the latest and best information about CHD so you can survive and even thrive despite it.

The goal of this book is to empower you with information about CHD. It can help you understand what CHD is, how to prevent it, how to find out if you have it, and finally, how to best treat it. By educating you about the risk factors for CHD, we hope to help you lower the risk for heart attack, stroke, and death for you and your loved ones. By telling you about the latest diagnostic and treatment techniques both for people with early and with advanced CHD, you and your doctor can make the best decisions to treat your disease. In addition, by giving you sound advice about lifestyle changes and medications, we give you the tools to stop—and possibly even reverse—your CHD.

People with CHD—or any illness for that matter—do best when they have a solid partnership with their health-care team.

The more informed you are, the better this team can work for you. After reading this book, it is our hope that you will be a more informed partner in protecting your heart.

There are no such things as incurables; there are only things [for] which man has not found a cure.
—Bernard M. Baruch
Presidential Advisor
1870-1965

1

What Is Coronary Heart Disease?

"You have coronary heart disease." When your doctor says those words to you or to someone you love, it's frightening and confusing. You probably have dozens of questions: What is coronary heart disease? Why did I get it? Do I need medication? Will I have to have surgery? Do I need to change my lifestyle? Hopefully, this book will answer these questions and many more.

Coronary heart disease (*CHD*), also called *coronary artery disease* (*CAD*) or *ischemic heart disease*, is a form of heart disease that's caused by narrowing of the coronary arteries that feed the heart. If you or someone you love has been diagnosed with CHD, it may help to know that you are not alone. In fact, CHD is the most common form of heart disease, affecting at least 12 million Americans. It is the single largest killer of both men and women in the United States, responsible for nearly a half million deaths each year, or about 1 out of every 5 deaths. CHD causes nearly all heart attacks (myocardial infarctions). Every 29 seconds, an American suffers a coronary event (a heart attack or fatal CHD), and every minute one of us will die from one. The American Heart Association estimates that this year alone, more than a million Americans will suffer from a new or recurrent coronary event, and nearly 40 percent of those will die from it.

Coronary heart disease isn't just an American problem. CHD is very common in other Westernized countries, too, such as many in Europe. Diseases of the heart and circulation such as heart attacks and stroke (a "brain attack") kill more people worldwide than any other cause. The World Health Organization estimates that as many as 30 percent of all deaths are caused by heart and circulation diseases like CHD.

The good news is that you don't have to become another CHD statistic. There is a lot you can do to reduce your risk of having a heart attack or dying from CHD. Sometimes just changing your lifestyle—following a heart-healthy diet, exercising regularly, and reducing the stress in your life—can prevent a heart attack or even reverse the narrowing in your arteries. There are a number of medications—and new ones being developed every day—that can help lower your heart attack risk. Surgical procedures such as angioplasty and stenting or bypass surgery can help compensate for blockages in your arteries and help keep your heart supplied with the blood it needs. By educating yourself about your treatment options with books such as this one and working closely with your doctor, you and your doctor can choose the best treatments that will enable you to live a long and healthy life.

The Circulatory System

The first step in taking charge of your CHD is to learn all you can about the disease. To understand what CHD is and how it affects your heart, you need to understand a little about your heart and how it works.

Your *circulatory system*, also called your *cardiovascular system*, is made up of the heart, the lungs, and blood vessels called *arteries* and *veins*. This system carries blood, food, and oxygen to every cell in the body. It also carries waste products away from the cells and out of the body. (A *cell* is the building block of every tissue and organ in the body.) Think of your circulatory system as a busy highway system composed of massive freeways and large streets that feed into smaller and smaller streets, and finally into tiny lanes and alleyways. This system is made up entirely of *one-way* streets. In our imaginary highway system, cars, or in this case, blood, can flow in only *one* direction. The one-way streets called arteries and *arterioles* (small arteries) carry blood enriched with

If the body's blood vessels were laid end to end, they'd cover about 60,000 miles—more than twice the circumference of the earth!

oxygen and nutrients *away* from the heart to the cells in the body. The one-way streets called veins and *venules* (small veins) carry blood loaded with waste products from the cells back *to* the heart.

Between these two one-way street systems are tiny blood vessels called *capillaries*. Almost too tiny to see and often thinner than a strand of hair, capillaries connect the smallest arteries with the smallest veins. They are the bridges that connect our two systems of one-way streets. The walls of these tiny capillaries are so thin that food and oxygen in the blood pass through them into the surrounding cells. These thin walls also allow waste products from the cells to pass into the capillaries. This enables the blood to carry waste from the cells to be removed by the kidneys, liver, and lungs.

If you can imagine a single drop of blood flowing through this system, it might look something like this. The blood droplet, full of oxygen and nutrients (fuel), is pumped out of the left side of the heart into the largest arteries. There it flows into progressively smaller arteries and finally into the capillaries, where it delivers its load of oxygen and food for the cells. At the same time, the blood picks up waste products from the cells and flows into tiny veins, then into larger and larger veins. Finally, the blood droplet arrives back at the right side of the heart, where it's pumped into the lungs to unload carbon dioxide, pick up a fresh supply of oxygen, and begin its circular journey again.

The Heart: An Amazing Pump

The heart is the pump that keeps the blood flowing around and around in an endless circle throughout the body. Think of it as the traffic cop that coordinates the flow of traffic throughout our highway system. The heart is a hollow muscle that weighs less than a pound and is about the size of a man's fist. Despite its small size, this amazing organ pumps an average of 100,000 times a day, pumping about 2,000 gallons of blood every day. If you live to be 70, your heart will beat more than 2.5 billion times.

Located in the center of the chest and protected by the breastbone and rib cage, the heart is actually a double pump that's divided into four chambers, two upper ones and two lower ones. A thin wall of muscle separates the left and right sides of the heart. The top chambers (*atriums* or *atria*) and lower chambers (*ventricles*) are connected by valves that act like one-way doors. These valves make sure blood flows only in

Exterior of the Heart

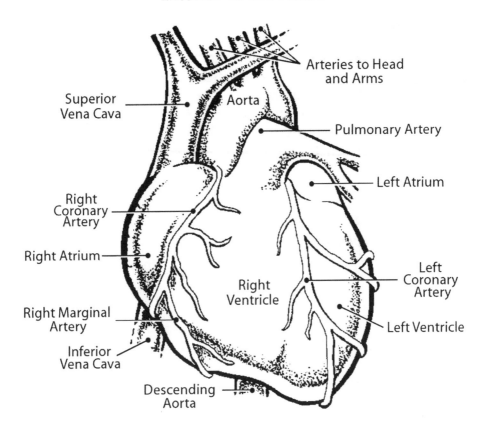

one direction. In the heart, the blood is pumped from the left and right atriums to the left and right ventricles. The right side of the heart sends blood to the lungs. The left side of the heart pumps blood out to the cells in the body.

Coronary Arteries

Just like other muscles in the body, the heart needs its own supply of blood and oxygen to work properly. Even though the heart pumps blood through its chambers, the heart itself receives no significant nourishment from this blood. There's a separate set of arteries that branch off the aorta (the main artery that receives blood from the left ventricle) that provide the heart's blood supply. These are called *coronary arteries*. The coronary arteries encircle the top and sides of the heart, bringing plenty of oxygen-rich blood to the heart. The two major coronary arteries are the *left coronary artery* and the *right coronary artery*. These vessels divide into many smaller coronary arteries that feed the heart.

Arteries are strong and elastic to withstand pressure as the heart pumps. Veins have valves to help blood return to the heart.

What Is Coronary Heart Disease?

Healthy coronary arteries have smooth, flexible walls that provide plenty of blood to the heart. However, over many years, these flexible walls can become progressively irritated and damaged by such substances as fats, cholesterol, calcium, cellular debris, and *platelets* (tiny cells responsible for blood clotting). When the walls of the arteries are damaged, these substances are able to "stick" to them. Coronary heart disease (CHD) occurs when these coronary arteries become narrowed and clogged.

This buildup inside the artery walls is a process called *atherosclerosis*, which produces a substance known as *plaque*. As it builds, plaque is a lot like the dirt, fat, and minerals that build up inside your home's plumbing. As the buildup becomes thicker, the flow through the pipes becomes less and less and may even completely stop. Similarly, when your heart doesn't get enough oxygen due to narrowed arteries, you may feel chest pressure or pain called *angina.* If the blood supply to part of the heart is completely cut off, the result is often a *heart attack.*

Everyone has a certain amount of atherosclerosis as they age. For many of us, atherosclerosis begins in childhood. Some people have a rapid increase in the buildup of atherosclerotic plaque after age 30. For others, plaque buildup doesn't become a problem until we're in our 50s or 60s.

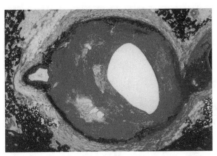

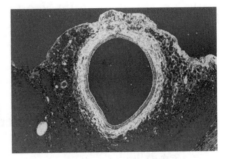

Plaque buildup obstructs the flow of blood through the artery. The white area, in the center, represents the only portion of the artery not blocked. *Custom Medical Stock Photo.*

An open artery, shown above, easily transports oxygenated blood away from the heart to other parts of the body. *Custom Medical Stock Photo.*

What Causes CHD?

We don't know for sure why atherosclerosis occurs or even how it begins, but there are several theories. Some medical experts believe the atherosclerotic buildup in the inner layers of the arteries may be caused by several conditions, including:

- Elevated levels of LDL cholesterol (low-density lipoprotein) and trigylcerides in the blood
- Low levels of HDL cholesterol (high-density lipoprotein)
- High blood pressure
- Tobacco smoke
- High blood sugar levels (diabetes mellitus)
- Inflammation

It's likely that more than one process is involved in the buildup of plaque. Many researchers believe that when excess fats combine with oxygen, they become trapped in the arterial wall. This attracts *white blood cells* which help prevent infection when tissue is damaged. Then substances called *prostaglandins,* which are involved in blood clotting and altering *tone* (firmness) within arteries, become active. Any injury to the artery wall, such as damage caused by smoking, can activate prostaglandins. The activated prostaglandins stimulate more plaque growth and narrow arteries and/or cause blood clots to form.

Regardless of how plaque forms, advanced plaque is made up mostly of living cells. In fact, about 85 percent of advanced plaque consists of cell debris, calcium, smooth muscle cells, connective tissue, and *foam cells* (white blood cells that have digested fat). About 15 percent of advanced plaque is made up of fatty deposits.

Once the plaque develops, plaque containing cells can be easily damaged. This can lead to blood clots forming on the outside of the plaque. Small clots can further damage other layers of the blood vessel wall and stimulate more plaque growth. Larger blood clots can partially or totally block the artery.

In addition to interfering with or totally blocking blood flow, plaque can hinder the artery's ability to dilate and contract. In order to respond to the body's ever-changing need for blood, the arteries need to be strong and elastic. For instance, when you exercise, your body needs more blood. The heart responds by pumping faster, and the arteries respond by expanding to accommodate the increased volume of blood coming from the heart. As the artery becomes narrowed and hard, that elasticity is lost. Arteries that have atherosclerotic plaque are more apt to *spasm* (temporarily narrow), causing even less blood to flow to the heart and possibly causing chest pain or heart attack.

2

Risk Factors for Coronary Heart Disease

You may be wondering why you developed coronary heart disease. We don't know exactly why some people develop CHD while others do not. We do know that certain traits or lifestyle habits put you more at risk. These are called *risk factors*. The more risk factors you have, the higher your chances of having a heart attack or stroke. Many of the risk factors for heart attack and stroke also tend to speed up the rate at which atherosclerotic plaque builds up. That's why it's important to understand and control the risk factors for CHD. By controlling your risk factors you may be able to:

- Slow down or even reverse the plaque building of atherosclerosis
- Help prevent a heart attack or stroke

According to the National Heart, Lung, and Blood Institute of the National Institutes of Health, having multiple risk factors for CHD doesn't just add to your risk, it multiplies it. If, for instance, you're a smoker who has high blood pressure and high blood cholesterol, your risk for CHD is eight times greater than someone with no risk factors. *Major risk factors* are those that studies have shown significantly contribute to cardiovascular disease. *Contributing risk factors* are associated with increased risk, but more research needs to confirm their contribution to CHD. Most risk factors for CHD can be changed. Others, such as increasing age, family history, your race or gender, cannot be changed.

Major CHD Risk Factors

Increasing Age

The older you are, the greater your risk for CHD, heart attack, and stroke. Four out of five people who die from CHD are 65 or older. If you're a man 45 years or older, you're at increased risk for heart attack or stroke. If you're a woman 55 years or older, or you've passed menopause, or you've had your ovaries removed, you're at increased risk.

The aging process itself is partly to blame for the increased risk for CHD, heart attack, and stroke. As we age, the connective tissues in our artery walls naturally become less flexible. This is called arteriosclerosis or "hardening of the arteries." This loss of flexibility in the arteries can cause the blood pressure to increase, which can damage arteries and lead to the buildup of plaque. Rising blood pressure and hardened arteries

Major CHD Risk Factors
- Increasing age
- Male gender
- Family history of heart disease
- Race
- Personal history of heart disease
- High blood cholesterol
- Smoking
- High blood pressure
- Overweight
- Physical inactivity
- Diabetes

Contributing CHD Risk Factors
- Stress
- Hormonal factors
- Birth control pills
- Excessive alcohol use
- Elevated homocysteine levels

can also make the heart have to work harder, which can cause the heart muscle to thicken and stiffen. Levels of blood cholesterol, another risk factor for CHD, also tend to rise with increasing age.

Male Gender

If you're a man, you have a greater chance of having a heart attack and having one earlier than women. This may be due to hormonal differences between men and women or other causes. Even when compared to postmenopausal women who have lost their gender protection against heart attack, men's rates of heart disease are greater.

Family History of Heart Disease

If members of your family suffered from heart disease, you have a greater risk for CHD, heart attack, and stroke. You have a greater risk if your father or brother had a heart attack before age 55 or if your mother or sister had one before age 65. You're also at increased risk if you have a relative who had a stroke.

Some people inherit genes that make them susceptible to the underlying causes of CHD such as diabetes, obesity, high blood cholesterol, or high blood pressure. For instance, diabetes or high blood pressure tends to run in some families. Other people may inherit risk factors such as *familial hypercholesterolemia*, a genetic disorder that makes them have excessively high LDL or "bad" blood cholesterol. For others, family lifestyle factors such as smoking, overeating, eating high-fat foods, and not exercising may contribute to increased risk.

Race

Some ethnic groups are at greater risk for CHD, heart attacks, and stroke. African Americans have higher rates of high blood pressure, a major risk factor for CHD. Mexican Americans, Native Americans, native Hawaiians, and some Asian Americans also have a higher risk for heart disease. Heart experts suspect higher risk among people in these groups may be related, in part, to their increased rates of obesity, diabetes, and cigarette smoking. Lack of access to good health care and economic disadvantages may also play a part in higher rates of heart disease and poorer prognosis among some groups.

In Japan, the incidence of CHD is lower than in Western countries. When people of Japanese ancestry immigrate to North America, their CHD risk climbs, but not as high as other Americans. This suggests that both genetics (race) and environment play a role in CHD.

Personal History of Heart Disease

If you have CHD, you're at increased risk for a heart attack or stroke. If you've already had a heart attack, you're at increased risk for having a second one.

High Blood Cholesterol

You've probably heard of blood cholesterol, including so-called good and bad cholesterol. You're likely confused about how it relates to CHD, heart attacks, and strokes. Having high blood cholesterol is one of the most important risk factors for CHD and subsequent heart attacks and strokes. However, it depends on the *type* of cholesterol. The higher your level of *LDL cholesterol* (low-density lipoprotein), the greater your risk.

When you have too much LDL cholesterol in your blood, the excess builds up on the walls of the coronary arteries. The opposite is true for HDL cholesterol (high-density lipoprotein). Having high HDL cholesterol protects against CHD; having low HDL cholesterol is a CHD risk factor.

Cholesterol is a waxy, fat-like substance that's found in every cell in the body. It's a useful substance that helps digest fats, strengthens cell membranes (linings), and makes some types of hormones and vitamins (e.g., vitamin D). However, too much cholesterol (*hyperlipidemia*) can be bad for you, causing artery-clogging plaque.

You get cholesterol in two ways: from the liver and from foods you eat. The liver produces all the cholesterol your body needs. Many of the foods we eat such as egg yolks, meats, poultry, and whole dairy products contain cholesterol. Eating too many of these foods can cause high blood cholesterol. As mentioned previously, you can also have high blood cholesterol if you have certain genetic factors such as familial hypercholesterolemia. Because high blood cholesterol is such a major risk factor, we'll talk more about it in chapter 3, "The Cholesterol-Coronary Heart Disease Connection."

Smoking

The American Heart Association calls smoking "the single most preventable cause of death in the United States." Thirty percent of all deaths from CHD in the United States are caused by smoking. In fact, smokers' risk of heart attack is *double* that of nonsmokers. Smokers who have heart attacks are twice as likely to die and die suddenly (within an hour) than nonsmokers. If you smoke and have other CHD risk factors, you significantly multiply your risk. For those with advanced atherosclerosis, smoking is especially dangerous.

According to a number of studies, including the famous Framingham Heart Study, smoking is a powerful risk factor for CHD and heart attack. When you smoke or are exposed to secondhand smoke:

- Blood pressure, heart rate, and the amount of blood pumped by the heart temporarily rise, which cause the heart to work harder.
- Arteries in the legs and arms constrict (narrow).
- Delicate tissues inside the arteries become damaged and are more subject to the buildup of artery-clogging plaque.
- Blood supply to the heart, especially in the tiny vessels supplying the heart muscle, decreases.
- Platelets, the clotting agents in blood, become stickier and tend to clump together. Smoking reduces clotting time and makes the blood thicker.
- Plaques that are already built up in the arteries can become destabilized. This promotes *rupture* (cracks in the inner walls of a blood vessel) and the formation of blood clots (*thrombi*) inside a blood vessel or chamber of the heart.
- "Bad" LDL cholesterol levels increase, and "good" HDL cholesterol levels in the blood decrease.

High Blood Pressure (HBP)

Blood pressure is the measurement of the force when the heart pumps blood into the arteries and out to the body *and* the

Blood Pressure Guidelines

Classification	Systolic Pressure (mmHg)	Diastolic Pressure (mmHg)
Optimal	< 120	< 80
Normal	< 130	< 85
High Normal	130-139	85-89
High Blood Pressure		
Stage 1	140-159	90-99
Stage 2	160-179	100-109
Stage 3	$\geq$ 180	$\geq$ 110

< = less than   > = greater than $\geq$ = equal to or greater than

force placed on the arteries as they resist the blood from the heart. It is written as two numbers—*systolic* (top number) and *diastolic* (bottom number)—expressed in millimeters of mercury (mmHg). The National Institutes of Health Joint National Committee on Blood Pressure has created categories for blood pressure. The higher your blood pressure, the greater your risk for CHD, heart attack, and other health problems.

When your blood pressure is too high (140/90 mmHg or higher), also called *hypertension*, your heart has to work harder. Over time, this can cause the heart muscle to become larger and thicker and may ultimately weaken the heart, making it unable to meet the body's need for blood and oxygen (*heart failure*).

High blood pressure (HBP) damages the arteries and arterioles, scarring them and making them hard and less elastic. It also speeds up the buildup of atherosclerotic plaque and may lead to heart attacks. As arteries become narrower, it becomes more likely that clots may form and block the blood supply completely.

If you have HBP and other CHD risk factors such as obesity, smoking, diabetes, and/or high blood cholesterol, your risk multiplies. HBP is also associated with stroke, kidney failure, and serious eye damage.

Overweight

Being overweight increases your risk for CHD and heart attack as well as for a number of other health problems. If you carry your excess weight around your waist (the so-called apple shape), your heart disease risk is even higher. Being overweight:

- Forces the heart to work harder
- Raises blood pressure
- Increases blood cholesterol and trigylcerides (a type of blood fat)
- Lowers "good" HDL blood cholesterol
- Increases the risk for developing diabetes, another risk factor for CHD

Physical Inactivity

If you're a couch potato, you're at risk for heart disease and heart attack. Heart experts have determined that being inactive is a major risk factor for heart disease/heart attack. The risk may be as high as six times the risk of heart disease as compared to those who are active.

If you don't exercise and you overeat, you may be putting yourself at even greater risk. Not exercising and overeating may cause you to become overweight, have high blood pressure and/or high blood cholesterol, and develop diabetes—all important risk factors for CHD and heart attack.

Diabetes

Diabetes mellitus is a problem with the body's metabolism, or energy-burning system. When you have diabetes, your body isn't able to produce and/or properly respond to the hormone *insulin*. Insulin allows your body to convert blood sugar (*glucose*) into energy. Diabetes is also a major risk factor for heart disease and heart attacks. Two-thirds of people with diabetes die from some form of heart or blood vessel disease.

Type 2 diabetes, or *adult-onset diabetes*, is the type that often develops around middle age. Being overweight and inactive are two risk factors that put you at risk for developing diabetes. Many people who have mild type 2 diabetes don't even know it for many years. Untreated, diabetes can cause a number of serious health problems, including blood vessel disease that can affect the eyes and kidneys.

Even when your diabetes is treated and you have your blood glucose levels under control, having diabetes significantly increases your risk for heart disease and stroke. One of the reasons for this may be that diabetes affects blood cholesterol and triglyceride levels (triglycerides are a type of blood fat associated with CHD). In addition, people with diabetes often have high blood pressure, another major risk factor for CHD and heart attacks.

Contributing CHD Risk Factors

The following risk factors are associated with CHD and heart attack, but additional research needs to be done to find out exactly *how* they contribute and *how much* they contribute to the CHD/heart attack equation.

Stress

All of us have stress in our lives and everyone reacts to stress a little differently. Some people are cool and calm most of the time. Stressful events don't seem to faze them much. Others have a "shorter fuse" and tend to overreact to the smallest stresses. While heart experts aren't all in agreement about the correlation between heart disease and how we react to stress, a growing body of evidence suggests that those who react more negatively to stress (for example, becoming angry or depressed) may be at greater risk for heart problems. A six-year study conducted at the University of North Carolina at Chapel Hill found those who were prone to anger were three times more likely to have a heart attack or sudden cardiac death than those who weren't anger-prone. At a recent annual meeting of the American College of Cardiology, researchers from Johns Hopkins reported similar results. They found that people who reacted to stress in a hot-tempered manner were nineteen times more likely to suffer *ischemia* (reduced blood flow to the heart), and their coronary arteries and other blood vessels stayed constricted for an abnormally long period of time.

We don't know if stress is an independent risk factor for CHD or if it simply affects other CHD risk factors such as high blood pressure. We do know that stress may cause a person to adopt unhealthful behaviors such as overeating or cigarette smoking that can contribute to heart disease.

Hormonal Factors

Sex hormones appear to affect one's risk for CHD and heart attacks. It's well known that men suffer more heart attacks and suffer them about ten years earlier than women. Female hormones tend to raise "good" HDL cholesterol and reduce "bad" LDL cholesterol. In contrast, male hormones do just the opposite.

A number of studies suggest that after menopause the loss of natural estrogen puts women at higher risk for CHD and heart attack. Women who undergo surgical menopause by the removal of the uterus and ovaries and who do not take replacement hormones have a dramatic rise in heart attack risk (similar to men's risk).

Birth Control Pills

Early forms of birth control pills often contained high doses of estrogen. While women's natural female hormones have a heart-protective effect, inexplicably, high estrogen-dose birth control pills do not. These birth control pills are associated with an increased risk for heart attack and stroke, especially among older women who smoke cigarettes. Newer pills contain less estrogen and therefore have a much lower risk.

Women who smoke and take birth control pills—even newer, lower-dose ones—are at higher risk for developing blood clots. After age 35, smoking and taking birth control pills increases heart attack risk even more.

Excessive Alcohol Use

We have all heard that drinking a small amount of alcohol may lower the risk of heart disease. However, drinking excessively (more than one drink per day for women, more than two drinks per day for men) increases heart disease risk. Drinking too much alcohol can increase blood pressure, a major risk factor for CHD and heart attack. Excessive drinking has been associated with irregular heartbeats and high triglycerides, a type of blood fat that may contribute to CHD. It can cause heart failure, a condition in which the heart is unable to pump enough blood to supply all the parts of the body. Alcohol also contributes to obesity, another major CHD risk factor.

Elevated Homocysteine Levels

Homocysteine is an *amino acid,* or protein building block. It is a natural by-product of the body's breakdown of protein. We also know that homocysteine is necessary for the production of two other amino acids, *cysteine* and *methionine.* Low intakes of folate, vitamin B_6, and vitamin B_{12} are associated with higher levels of homocysteine.

For more than thirty years, researchers have speculated that elevated levels of homocysteine may be a cause of atherosclerosis. Research in the past ten years confirms that elevated levels of homocysteine is a risk factor for CHD. Thirty percent of the heart patients in the Framingham Heart Study had elevated levels of homocysteine.

We aren't sure how elevated levels of homocysteine contribute to heart disease. One theory suggests that high levels of homocysteine causes blood vessel walls to narrow. Homocysteine may also encourage the development of blood clots by interfering with a natural anticoagulant, *protein C.*

3

The Cholesterol-Coronary Heart Disease Connection

Numerous research studies have established that abnormalities in cholesterol, particularly high LDL cholesterol and low HDL cholesterol, play a major role in the development of CHD and heart attacks. Cholesterol is one of the major components of artery-clogging plaque, so it's important to understand more about cholesterol and its relationship to heart disease.

As mentioned before, the waxy, fat-like substance cholesterol is necessary for life. However, the body needs only a small amount of cholesterol. The liver produces about 1,000 milligrams of cholesterol every day, or about 80 percent of your blood cholesterol. That's all the cholesterol your body really needs.

We also get cholesterol from foods that come from animals such as meats, poultry, fish, egg yolks, and whole milk products. About 20 percent of our blood cholesterol comes from dietary cholesterol. The amount of fat and cholesterol you eat can influence all your blood fats, including blood cholesterol levels.

The problem comes when there's too much cholesterol circulating in the bloodstream. As you know by now, excess cholesterol can lead to atherosclerosis, the plaque-building process that narrows arteries throughout the body and can lead to chest pain, heart attack, or stroke.

Types of Cholesterol

Everyone knows that oil and water do not mix. The same is true for cholesterol and blood. Cholesterol cannot dissolve in blood. To enable cholesterol to travel through the blood, the body coats cholesterol with proteins called *apoproteins.* Once combined with the protein, a complex called a *lipoprotein* is formed. These protein carriers transport cholesterol and triglycerides (another type of blood fat) through the bloodstream. There are several different types of lipoprotein. Each affects CHD and heart attack risk differently.

More than half of all Americans have total cholesterol levels higher than 200 mg/dL, putting them at increased risk for CHD and heart attack.

Low-Density Lipoprotein (LDL) Cholesterol

This type of lipoprotein is called "bad" cholesterol because it is the main source of cholesterol in the blood and one of the major culprits in the buildup of atherosclerotic plaque. (Remember that LDL is the "bad" cholesterol by associating the L with "lousy.") LDL cholesterol carries some 60 to 70 percent of the body's circulating cholesterol.

As LDL cholesterol circulates through the bloodstream, the body uses some of it for jobs like building cells. Some of the cholesterol returns to the liver. However, when there is too much LDL cholesterol circulating in the blood, it can slowly build up on the walls of the coronary arteries. The more LDL cholesterol you have in your blood, the higher your risk for CHD and heart attack.

High-Density Lipoprotein (HDL) Cholesterol

This is the so-called good cholesterol. High-density lipoprotein packages, which contain mostly protein, carry anywhere from 20 to 30 percent of the cholesterol in the blood. HDL cholesterol is considered "good" because it acts like a trash collector, picking up excess cholesterol from the artery walls and sending it to the liver for disposal. Thus, HDL cholesterol slows plaque growth and may reverse the plaque-building process. The higher your level of HDL, the lower your risk of heart disease and heart attack. Conversely, low levels of HDL increase your risk for CHD and heart attack.

Very Low-Density Lipoprotein (VLDL) Cholesterol

The largest of the lipoproteins, VLDL contains about 15 percent of the blood's cholesterol and most of the triglycerides. A significant amount of VLDL is converted to LDL cholesterol. Consequently, some types of VLDL cholesterol may contribute to plaque building.

Triglycerides

Triglycerides are another type of blood fat. Most of the body's fat is stored as triglycerides in fat tissue. A small portion of triglycerides circulate in the blood. Triglyceride levels in the blood are related to how much and what kind of dietary fat and carbohydrates (sugar and starches) and how much alcohol you consume. Triglyceride levels are also influenced by genetics.

Heart experts believe that excessive levels of triglycerides may contribute to the fatty deposits that obstruct blood flow and increase the risk for heart attack.

A twenty-year study recently published in *Circulation* found that people with elevated triglycerides have a greater risk of dying from a heart attack, even if their blood cholesterol is normal.

The Problem of Unstable Plaques

As excess cholesterol travels in the blood, it is taken up by special cells in the artery walls. This creates "lumps" in the artery walls that are covered over or encapsulated by fibrous scar-tissue. Some of these so-called stable plaques become quite large and dramatically narrow or even totally block arteries. When these large blockages reduce the amount of blood getting to the heart, they can cause the chest pain, or angina.

It is the smaller, *unstable plaques* which are thinly or not entirely covered over by scar tissue that pose the biggest threat for heart attacks. These plaques are loaded with cholesterol and have a tendency to rupture easily. When these unstable plaques burst into the artery channel (*lumen*), they release their cholesterol back into the local bloodstream. The body responds by triggering a blood clot inside the artery to repair the perceived damage to the inner artery wall. This blood clot may totally block the artery, stopping blood flow and causing a heart attack. The area of the heart that doesn't receive blood starts to die within twenty minutes, permanently damaging the heart muscle. Even if the clot doesn't cause a heart attack, it can cause electrical disturbances that interfere with the heart's rhythm (*arrhythmias*). This can lead to cardiac arrest (sudden stopping of the heart) and death.

Reducing the amount of cholesterol in the blood can help lower the amount of cholesterol in plaques, making them more stable and less likely to burst and trigger a heart attack. Even in people who have already had a heart attack, lowering cholesterol can lower the chance of having another heart attack in the future.

What Constitutes High Cholesterol?

Doctors measure blood levels of total cholesterol, HDL and LDL cholesterol, and triglycerides to assess the risk of atherosclerosis and heart attack. Previously, heart experts recommended that people without heart disease have their total cholesterol and HDL cholesterol tested every five years.

Cholesterol Guidelines for Adults (without CHD)

	Optimal	Desirable	Borderline High	High	Very High
Total Cholesterol		< 200 mg/dL	201-239 mg/dL	≥ 240 mg/dL	
HDL Cholesterol		> 40 mg/dL+		≥ 60 mg/dL	
LDL Cholesterol	< 100 mg/dL	< 130 mg/dL	130-159 mg/dL	160-189 mg/dL	≥ 190 mg/dL
Triglycerides		< 150 mg/dL	150-199 mg/dL	200-499 mg/dL	500 mg/dL

< = less than   > = greater than   ≥ = equal to or greater than

However, we now recognize that because LDL is a major cause of CHD, it is also important to measure LDL.

According to guidelines from the National Heart, Lung, and Blood Institute's National Cholesterol Education Program Expert Panel (NCEP), all adults over age 20 should have their total cholesterol, HDL and LDL cholesterol, and triglyceride levels checked at least once every five years. Doctors call this test a *lipoprotein* or *lipid profile*.

Factors in High Cholesterol

In most cases, there is no single cause of high blood cholesterol. Your blood cholesterol level may certainly be affected by your diet. But it may also be affected by how quickly your body makes LDL cholesterol and how rapidly it gets rid of it.

Genetics

Genes you inherit from your family can influence how rapidly your body makes LDL cholesterol and how efficiently it's removed. Your liver might produce too many VLDL particles or two few HDL particles, making you prone to high cholesterol.

Some people—approximately 1 in 500—have familial hypercholesterolemia, an inherited disorder that causes cholesterol levels to be extremely high (350 to 500 mg/dL). Even if you don't have an

---

Factors in High Cholesterol

- Genetics
- Diet
- Calorie balance and your weight
- Physical activity
- Age
- Menopause
- Smoking
- Diabetes
- Stress

31

inherited cholesterol disorder, your genetics influence your cholesterol levels.

Diet

What you eat influences your blood cholesterol levels too. How much *saturated fat* (a type of fat that comes mostly in foods from animals such as meat, egg yolks, and dairy products) and dietary cholesterol you eat can raise or lower your cholesterol levels.

Calorie Balance and Your Weight

Calorie balance refers to the number of calories you take in versus the number of calories you burn each day. When you take in more calories than you burn, you gain weight. Excess weight tends to increase LDL cholesterol levels. When your extra pounds are around your waist, your risk for heart disease is even greater. Losing weight can lower LDL cholesterol levels, raise "good" HDL cholesterol, and reduce triglyceride levels.

Physical Activity

Inactivity can negatively influence your blood cholesterol levels. Regular physical activity can decrease "bad" VLDL cholesterol, raise "good" HDL cholesterol levels, and, in some people, even lower "bad" LDL cholesterol levels.

Age

As men and women get older, their blood cholesterol levels tend to rise. This rise usually levels off at about 60 to 65 years of age.

Menopause

Women's total blood cholesterol levels tend to be lower than those for men of the same age. However, after menopause, women's LDL cholesterol increases and their HDL cholesterol tends to decrease. Some authorities believe this change in cholesterol levels may be why women's risk of heart disease rises sharply after menopause.

Smoking

In addition to damaging blood vessel walls and making them more susceptible to the development of atherosclerotic plaque, smoking can lower "good" HDL cholesterol levels by as much as 15 percent.

Diabetes

In many people, diabetes can increase triglycerides and decrease "good" HDL cholesterol levels.

Stress

While it's hard to pin down the impact of stress in heart disease, some studies indicate that over a long period of time stress raises blood cholesterol levels. It's unclear whether this rise is due to the direct effect stress has on the body's chemistry, or whether it's because stress may influence people to indulge in behaviors such as smoking and overeating that are risky for the heart.

If your doctor prescribes cholesterol-lowering medication, you will also need to:

- Follow a cholesterol-lowering diet
- Be physically active (as recommended by your doctor)
- Lose excess weight if you're overweight
- Stop smoking
- Control your high blood pressure and diabetes

High Cholesterol: A Modifiable Risk Factor

In this chapter, we've seen how high cholesterol—especially high LDL cholesterol—increases your risk for CHD and heart attack. That's the bad news. The good news is that high cholesterol is a risk factor you can do something about. A number of studies have shown that lowering total cholesterol and LDL cholesterol reduces CHD risk. A large study called the Scandinavian Simvastatin Survival Study showed that lowering cholesterol levels can prevent heart attacks and reduce death in men and women who already have heart disease. The study's subjects reduced their total cholesterol levels by 25 percent and LDL cholesterol levels by 35 percent with medication. By doing so, they reduced deaths from heart disease by 42 percent, the chance of having a nonfatal heart attack by 37 percent, and the need for bypass surgery or angioplasty by 37 percent.

This study and many others point to the positive benefits of lowering total and LDL cholesterol levels. We'll talk more about how you can reduce your cholesterol in chapters 7 and 9.

4

Symptoms of Coronary Heart Disease

Symptoms are subjective changes in the way the body feels that may signal illness or disease. A symptom isn't the disease itself, but a feeling or complaint that something is wrong. You may have coronary heart disease and not even know it. Especially in the early stages of CHD, you may have no symptoms at all. You feel fine, unaware that there's a silent time bomb ticking away inside your coronary arteries. As the arteries become narrower and the heart begins to have less and less blood and oxygen available to it, you may experience shortness of breath or angina—periodic pain, tightness, or pressure in the chest. Other people may have no symptoms. Their first indication that they have CHD is a potentially deadly heart attack.

Silent Ischemia

When there is a temporary shortage of blood and oxygen to the heart without any symptoms, it's called *silent ischemia*. It can occur when a coronary artery is narrowed by atherosclerotic plaque, or spasm, or a combination of the two. The problem with silent ischemia is that there's no pain, no discomfort, no warning—until there's a heart attack. It's like a smoke detector that's been disconnected—it prevents the alarm being sounded when a fire breaks out.

Angina

Pressure, pain, and/or tightness in the chest is the symptom most commonly associated with CHD. It occurs when the heart doesn't receive enough blood and oxygen.

Angina or *angina pectoris* is often a recurring pain or discomfort in the chest that occurs when part of the heart doesn't get enough blood. People often describe angina as pressure, squeezing, burning, tightness, or heaviness. Most commonly the discomfort is felt under the breastbone. However, sometimes people feel discomfort in the shoulders, arms, neck, jaws, or back. Some people also experience numbness in the shoulders, arms, or wrists.

Angina usually lasts a few minutes—typically no more than 5 to 15 minutes. Things that trigger angina include: exertion or physical stress (times when the heart's demand for oxygen increases), eating a heavy meal, exposure to extreme heat or cold, drinking alcohol, and cigarette smoking. It may be relieved within a few minutes by stopping the stressful activity.

Angina is *not* a heart attack. During angina, blood flow to the heart is less than the heart needs at the time. This reduction causes the discomfort. Angina attacks usually do not permanently damage the heart muscle. In contrast, during a heart attack, blood flow to part of the heart is completely (or nearly) blocked. The pain that results is usually more severe and lasts longer, and the damage to the heart muscle may be serious and is permanent.

But chest pain may also be caused by other serious heart and circulatory problems: pericarditis, dissection of the aorta, or pulmonary embolism.

Pericarditis is an inflammation of the *pericardium,* the fibrous outer sac that surrounds the heart. The chest pain it causes is usually sharp, even knife-like. It's made worse by taking a deep breath or lying down and gets better when you lean forward.

Dissection of the aorta is a tearing of the inner lining of the major artery that leads away from the heart. The pain, often described as a tearing sensation, can be excruciating.

A *pulmonary embolism* is a blood clot in the lung. The pain is located in the chest and typically gets worse when you take a deep breath, or it may cause chest heaviness that's identical to angina. Both angina and pulmonary emboli may cause some degree of breathlessness.

Non-heart problems may also cause pain and discomfort similar to angina. For instance, gallbladder disease or inflammation of the esophagus from the reflux of stomach acid often referred to as GERD (gastroeseophageal reflux disease) both cause chest pain. Problems in the joints, nerves, or chest wall can also cause angina-like pain.

Types of Angina

We classify angina as stable or unstable. If you have *stable angina,* you probably experience chest discomfort when you overexert. The pain is relatively predictable and, almost any time you overexert, the pain comes back. For instance, you may feel chest pain and tightness when you perform heavy labor such as shoveling snow or during times of emotional stress.

Over time, you probably learn to identify what brings on your angina attacks.

Unstable angina is less predictable. It includes:

- New chest pain or discomfort that may come on suddenly during activities that never caused problems before
- A changing pattern of stable angina (pain occurring at lower levels of activity, more often, or more severely)
- Chest pain that occurs at rest or that wakes one from sleep

Unstable angina is more dangerous because it carries a higher risk of heart attack. Although both stable and unstable angina are caused by the atherosclerotic plaques of CHD, the plaque in unstable angina is more prone to rupture on the inner surface of the artery. When this happens, the body forms a blood clot to repair the damage. If the clot is large enough, it may block blood flow and cause a heart attack. Unstable angina can also cause severe heart rhythm problems or sudden cardiac death, in which the heart muscle simply stops functioning.

A third, less common type of angina is called *variant* or *Prinzmetal's angina.* In this form of angina, the muscle fibers surrounding the coronary arteries go into spasm. This causes the blood vessel to become very narrow or even close off completely. About 65 percent of people who suffer variant angina have severe coronary atherosclerotic plaque in at least one major coronary vessel. The spasm usually occurs very close to the artery blockage. Variant angina attacks often occur without exertion or other apparent cause. Other times the attacks may be brought on by stress, exposure to cold, or cigarette smoking. Variant angina attacks are usually severe and last only a short time. They often occur between midnight and 8:00 A.M., waking the person from sleep with the discomfort. During attacks, abnormal heart rhythms can cause the person to lose consciousness.

The Heart's Warning

Regardless of the type of angina you may have, it has the same cause: not enough oxygen getting to the heart due to atherosclerotic plaque. Angina is a warning from your heart. Angina may not indicate that you are about to have a heart attack. It does mean that you have underlying CHD and that you may be at increased risk for heart attack. If you experience angina:

Don't ignore it. Angina is your body's cry for help. See your doctor *immediately* for evaluation. *Don't wait a few days or a few weeks for an appointment to address the symptoms.* Once your condition is properly diagnosed, your doctor can prescribe lifestyle changes, medication, or medical procedures such as angioplasty to relieve your discomfort.

Know what angina is. Not all chest pain is angina. The pain is probably *not* angina if:

- It lasts for less than 30 seconds
- Taking a deep breath relieves it
- It goes away after drinking a glass of water
- It disappears if you change body positions
- It's localized on the surface of your chest and you can reproduce it by touching a particular spot

If you have any doubt, see your doctor. Remember, it's better to have the problem checked out early.

Learn the pattern of your angina. Once your doctor has evaluated and treated your condition, try to learn what brings on and what relieves attacks. Pay attention to what your angina attacks feel like, how long episodes usually last, and how medication affects them.

Watch for changes. When the pattern of angina changes, the risk of heart attack increases for days or even weeks. See your doctor right away if your angina:

Take angina seriously, especially if you smoke, are overweight, have a family history of heart disease, have high cholesterol, are diabetic, or have high blood pressure.

- Becomes more frequent
- Lasts longer
- Occurs at rest

Know the symptoms of a heart attack. See the list of symptoms in this chapter and commit it to memory. Call for emergency medical help (911 in most areas) immediately if the pattern of your angina changes sharply or if you have any symptoms of heart attack.

Heart Attack

Doctors call it a *coronary attack* or *myocardial infarction (MI)*. Other names for heart attack include *coronary occlusion* or *coronary thrombosis*. Basically, all these mean the same thing to someone who suffers a heart attack.

A heart attack occurs when the blood supply to part of the heart is severely reduced or completely blocked. This occurs when one of the coronary arteries supplying the heart becomes severely narrowed or blocked, usually from a combination of too much atherosclerotic plaque and a blood clot. Typically, when plaque tears or ruptures, the cholesterol core of the plaque is exposed to circulating blood cells (platelets). In response, the body forms a blood clot. If this blood clot severely restricts or blocks the blood supply to part of the heart, a heart attack can occur.

If heart cells are denied blood and oxygen for a prolonged period of time, they suffer irreversible injury and begin to die. Depending on how much of the heart is damaged, it can cause the heart to be unable to pump enough blood to the body (heart failure) or cause death.

Heart attacks can also occur when a coronary artery temporarily goes into spasm. This can reduce or even stop blood flow to part of the heart, especially if the coronary artery is already narrowed by atherosclerotic plaque. Many factors contribute to spasm, including the local release of chemical substances that may trigger spasm and the sensitivity of the artery to contract. Both normal and diseased arteries may develop spasm. If the spasm is severe enough, a heart attack can result.

Common Heart Attack Symptoms:

- Uncomfortable pressure, tightness, fullness, squeezing, or pain in the center of the chest
- Pain that lasts more than a few minutes (30 minutes to several hours) or goes away and comes back
- Pain that spreads to the shoulders, neck, or arms
- Light-headedness or fainting
- Nausea
- Profuse sweating
- Shortness of breath

Less Typical Signs of a Heart Attack

Not everyone experiences a heart attack the same way. Even if you've had one or more heart attacks, the next heart attack may feel different. Some people feel the classic, heavy heart-attack chest pain. People often describe it as a "vice squeezing my chest." Others may have only a vague sense of discomfort, indigestion, breathlessness, and/or dizziness. People who have diabetes, women, and people over the age of 75 often have symptoms that are less typical.

- Vague chest pain
- Stomach or abdominal pain
- Nausea or dizziness, without chest pain
- Shortness of breath or difficulty breathing, without chest pain
- Anxiety without obvious cause, impending sense of doom
- Weakness or fatigue
- Erratic heartbeating
- Cold sweating
- Paleness
- Frequent angina not caused by exertion
- Dry mouth or cough, usually with breathlessness

Immediate Medical Care is Critical

With heart attacks, time is critical. The longer the artery is blocked, the more damage to the heart muscle and the greater the risk of permanent disability or even death. Additionally, a heart attack can cause the electrical signals of the heart that regulate its rhythm and pumping to become scrambled. Instead of pumping in a synchronized fashion, the heart twitches errati-cally (*ventricular fibrillation*) and becomes unable to pump blood. If ventricular fibrillation lasts longer than a few minutes, it can cause death.

Many people mistake the symptoms of a heart attack for indigestion or stress. They delay getting to the hospital. This is a dangerous and often fatal mistake. *Anyone who experiences a heart attack should be rushed to the nearest hospital* (they should *not* drive themselves).

If you get to an emergency room fast, doctors can use a variety of techniques and medications to help restore blood flow to the part of the heart that is damaged during the heart attack. Called *reperfusion therapy*, this may involve clot-dissolving medications, balloon angioplasty (and stenting), or surgery. Restoring the heart's blood flow is vitally important because damage to even less than 10 percent of the ventricle muscle decreases the amount of blood your heart can pump with each beat. If 25 percent or more of the heart muscle is damaged, your heart can enlarge and be unable to pump adequately (heart failure). When 40 percent or more of the heart muscle is damaged, shock or death may result. *The sooner the doctors can use reperfusion techniques on your heart, the more likely you'll survive.* In fact, one study by the University of Washington showed that three-quarters of people survived heart attacks with little or no heart damage when they received clot-dissolving therapy within 70 minutes of the beginning of

Sixty percent of people who die of a heart attack die within the first hour. Get help fast. Time is critical in a heart attack.

symptoms. Better blood thinners are continuing to improve these results.

The results are even better when there's an experienced cardiologist available at the hospital to perform direct angioplasty (a procedure that opens the arteries) and stenting (propping open the arteries with fine wire mesh). This approach can reduce death rates from heart attacks to less than 5 percent at a six-month follow-up. We'll talk more about these two procedures in chapter 8.

Suggestions for Surviving a Heart Attack:

- Keep a list of emergency rescue numbers handy. Call 911 or other emergency medical number immediately if you experience symptoms.
- Know which medical centers offer 24-hour cardiac care and which one is closest to your home and office.
- Know and recognize the symptoms of heart attack. About half of all heart attack victims have warning signs hours, days, or even weeks before an attack. Be aware that not all heart attacks involve the classic crushing chest pain.
- Chew one regular-strength aspirin. It will help break up clots if you're having a heart attack. If you're not, it likely will not hurt you. When taken during a heart attack, aspirin can decrease death rates by about 25 percent. Chewing the aspirin speeds its absorption.
- If your doctor has given you nitroglycerine tablets, place one under your tongue when symptoms begin. Repeat every five minutes for a total of three doses. (Do *not* take nitroglycerine if your doctor hasn't

prescribed it for you or if you feel dizzy, unless you're
directly supervised by a health-care professional.
Taking nitroglycerine for some types of heart
conditions can be dangerous. Do NOT take
nitroglycerine if you took sildenafil—*Viagra* within 24
hours.)

- If you can't get ambulance service, have someone
  drive you (don't drive yourself) to the nearest
  emergency medical facility.

- Have someone close to you trained in *cardiopulmonary
  resuscitation* (*CPR*). You may need it if your heart
  stops beating. CPR can help parts of your body receive
  oxygen until emergency medical help arrives.

Sudden Cardiac Death

Sudden cardiac death (*SCD*) is the most dramatic event of
CHD. In fact, it's the most common reason people die from
CHD. SCD is the abrupt, total loss
of heart function (*cardiac arrest*) in
someone with or without diag-
nosed heart disease. Death is unexpected. About half of all
deaths from atherosclerosis are from SCD.

> *Chewing aspirin during a heart
> attack can save your life.*

People who die from SCD almost always have underlying
heart disease. Most often, it is atherosclerosis. In about 90
percent of those who die from SCD, two or more major
coronary arteries are narrowed by atherosclerotic plaque.
Two-thirds of SCD victims have heart damage from previous
heart attacks. The first six months following a heart attack is a
high-risk time for people to die from SCD.

SCD has the same risk factors as CHD. Strategies to reduce risk factors for CHD and reduce/prevent atherosclerosis can help reduce the risk of dying from SCD.

5

Women and Coronary Heart Disease

Many women believe that coronary heart disease is "a man's problem." Nothing could be further from the truth. Heart disease (especially CHD) and stroke are the leading causes of death for women in the United States and in most developed countries. Every year, heart disease and stroke kills more than half a million women in this country, nearly twice as many as from all forms of cancer, including breast cancer. In fact, twice as many women die from heart disease as from breast cancer. The risk is even greater for minority women. The rate of death for black women from heart disease is 69 percent higher than for white women. They're more likely to die of a heart attack before menopause, too.

Unfortunately, most women are not aware of their risk for heart disease. A recent poll conducted for the American Heart Association found that most women do not recognize that heart disease is women's leading health problem and their number one cause of death today. In fact, fewer than 1 in 10 women believe heart disease is their greatest health threat.

Although CHD is the number one cause of death for women, a woman's first clue might be a full-blown, potentially fatal heart attack (or stroke if the blockage occurs in the brain). That's because the artery-clogging plaque building of athero-sclerosis is invisible. Over a lifetime, plaque deposits build silently. Two-thirds of women who die of a heart attack have no prior symptoms, compared to only half of men.

CHD isn't just a disease of older women. Certainly, women over 65 are most vulnerable to CHD. However, middle-aged women between 45 and 64 are at risk, too. One in nine American women in this age group show signs of CHD.

Medical Community Responds Differently

While women don't recognize the threat CHD poses, health experts have also been slow to recognize and respond to the problem of women and heart disease. Many of the studies conducted on heart disease have used male subjects. Only in the last few years have studies taken place that will clarify the sex differences in how heart disease manifests itself. The results of this research will improve diagnostic and treatment strategies for women.

In a survey of nearly 30,000 office visits, the Centers for Disease Control and Prevention found that doctors are less likely to provide women than men with information about heart-healthy nutrition, exercise, and weight reduction. This is disturbing news considering that:

- Obesity is increasing
- Approximately 25 percent of women report they get no regular physical activity
- Approximately 52 percent of women older than 45 have elevated blood pressure

- Nearly 40 percent of women 55 and older have elevated blood cholesterol levels
- Smoking rates for women are declining less than for men

Women are also less likely than men to get the right diagnosis and treatment for CHD. The American Heart Association concluded that both women and their doctors often attribute chest pains to non-heart causes, resulting in dangerous misdiagnoses. Part of this may be due to the fact that women are more apt to have subtle, atypical heart attack symptoms. While some women have the classic heart attack chest pain that radiates to the shoulders, neck, or arms, many have less typical chest discomfort or abdominal pain, difficulty breathing, and other less recognizable symptoms.

Some diagnostic tests such as the exercise stress test (ECG stress test) are less accurate for women, which may cause doctors to avoid using them. For instance, in young healthy women, the exercise stress test may give a false positive result. Routine treadmill tests may not pick up single-vessel heart disease, a more common type of CHD found in younger women. By delaying the diagnosis, the disease progresses untreated. Because women tend to develop and seek help for CHD later in life, diagnosis may also be hindered by the presence of other age-related diseases such as arthritis and osteoporosis.

Higher Death Rates in Women

When women do have heart attacks, they are more likely to die from them than men. One study published in the *New*

England Journal of Medicine found that women had higher heart attack death rates during hospitalization (16.7 percent for women versus 11.5 percent for men). Since the advent of reperfusion strategies (opening the heart attack related arteries) the mortality rates have declined for both men and women. Statistics from the National Heart, Lung, and Blood Institute and from the Framingham Heart Study reveal that more women who have heart attacks die within a year than men. This may be due, in part, to the fact that women tend avoid or delay seeking medical attention for their symptoms, perhaps due to lack of awareness. Women also have heart attacks later in life. Age and the more advanced stage of CHD limit a woman's treatment options and may increase her risk of death.

Women may also die more often from heart attacks because they receive less aggressive aftercare than men. A recent national survey found that women are less likely than men to enroll in cardiac rehabilitation programs following a heart attack or bypass surgery. Those involved in cardiac rehab programs are more likely to receive treatment for CHD risk factors. It may be that women, who are trained in North American culture to be caregivers for others, are less willing to care for themselves.

Mary was a 52-year-old teacher who felt fine, but had a strong family history of heart disease. Her father died at 46 of a heart attack. Her sister had a minor heart attack. Her brother, who had no symptoms, had a diagnostic test called an EBT (electron beam tomography) that measures the calcium in plaque deposits attached to artery walls and correlates it with heart disease risk. The higher the EBT calcium score, the greater the risk for heart attack. Mary's brother's calcium score was abnormally high. His doctor ordered a nuclear stress test, which was also abnormal, and his catheterization showed he had critical CHD. The cardiac surgeon performed a successful double-bypass. Worried that Mary might be next in the family line of heart disease, her brother asked Mary to get a cardiac evaluation.

Mary wasn't really worried. After all, she'd stopped smoking 10 years earlier and her cholesterol was in the low 200s. To ease her brother's mind, Mary finally asked her doctor for a nuclear stress test. The doctor resisted, believing that Mary didn't really need such a test. After Mary went in for an EBT that showed she had a high amount of calcium in her coronaries, the doctor reluctantly agreed to order a nuclear stress test for her. She was told that the test did show a minor defect, but that it was likely just breast tissue, not a coronary blockage. The doctor told her they'd repeat the test in one year. But now Mary was worried. She insisted on a catheterization, which showed critical narrowing in her coronary arteries (though she had no symptoms). Mary underwent a successful four-vessel bypass and is now back to school teaching.

Risk Factors for CHD in Women

Physiologically, men and women are different. So it shouldn't surprise us that CHD develops a bit differently in women and men. Some of the risk factors for CHD impact women differently than men.

Cigarette Smoking

A large 12-year study from Norway recently published in *Circulation* concluded that smoking poses greater dangers to women's hearts than to men's. Women who smoke 20 cigarettes or more per day are 6 times more likely to have a heart attack than women who never smoked. For men, the risk was 2.8 times greater when compared to non-smoking males. Why the difference? Cigarette smoking targets two of women's "natural protectors"—estrogen and higher amounts of "good" HDL cholesterol circulating in the blood. Researchers speculate that cigarette smoking may cause an "antiestrogenic effect" and lower HDL more in women than in men.

Women who smoke and take birth control pills are at even greater risk. Taking birth control pills and smoking increase a woman's risk of heart attack by as much as 39 times compared with women who don't smoke or take birth control pills.

Increasing Age

Compared with men, women's risk of heart disease is relatively low until menopause. The female hormone estrogen may have a protective effect by raising a woman's "good" HDL cholesterol and lowering "bad" LDL cholesterol. However, after menopause and the subsequent decrease in estrogen, a woman's risk of heart attack rises. At age 65, a woman's risk for heart attack is nearly that of men's.

Diabetes

Diabetes mellitus occurs when the body keeps too much glucose (sugar) in the bloodstream. The disease is a major risk factor for CHD and heart attack for both men and women, but it impacts women's risk even more dramatically. Having diabetes increases a woman's CHD risk by three to seven times compared with a twofold to threefold increase in men. This may be because diabetes in women has an especially negative effect on blood fats and blood pressure.

Cholesterol/Triglycerides

Total cholesterol levels are not as strong an indicator of heart disease for women as for men. For women, it appears that HDL levels are more important. Low levels of "good" HDL cholesterol are a reliable indicator of CHD in women. Low HDL levels appear to be a greater risk for CHD and heart attack for women older than 65 than in men of the same age. Some heart disease experts suggest that the national guideline of HDL levels of less than 35 mg/dL as an independent risk factor for CHD may be too low for women. They suggest 45 mg/dL or even higher HDL is a better standard.

In addition, women's trigylceride levels appear to have more influence in women's heart health. Women with trigylcerides higher than 190 mg/dL have a greater heart disease risk. Men's risk doesn't increase until triglycerides reach 400 mg/dL.

Weight

Being overweight contributes to increased risks for CHD and heart attacks for both men and women. However, when women accumulate their extra pounds around the waist, they are more subject to high blood pressure and insulin resistance, a precursor to diabetes.

CHD and Hormone Replacement Therapy (HRT)

Estrogen is a female hormone made primarily by a woman's ovaries. Estrogen helps keep women's bones strong and protects against heart disease. As women approach menopause, their level of estrogen drops and their risk for heart attack and stroke rises slowly. Women who undergo *surgical menopause* (removal of the ovaries) and who don't take estrogen replacement experience a sharp rise in the risk of heart attack and stroke. (A woman who undergoes *partial hysterectomy*—removal of the uterus, leaving at least one ovary— retains her hormonal protection.)

For many years, women and their doctors believed that *hormone replacement therapy* or *HRT* (given in pills or patches that contain estrogen or the combination of hormones, estrogen-progestin) provided postmenopausal women with protection against heart disease and heart attacks. New research from the large-scale Heart and Estrogen Replacement Study (HERS) found that HRT provides no protective heart benefit for women with heart disease. Additionally, the Estrogen Replacement and Atherosclerosis (ERA) Trial found HRT did not slow the progression of atherosclerosis in women with heart disease or blood vessel disease.

The American Heart Association advises doctors against prescribing HRT for the sole purpose of preventing heart attacks and strokes in women with heart disease. Instead, they recommend women with heart disease reduce their risk of heart attack and stroke by making lifestyles changes such as quitting smoking, losing weight, and exercising regularly. These are considered first-line CHD therapies. Medications to reduce high cholesterol and/or high blood pressure can also help lower risk.

There is evidence that statin medications, which lower cholesterol, are underprescribed in women and could help lower cholesterol levels better than hormone replacement therapy.

Population studies in the past have indicated that HRT reduces heart attacks in healthy women, those without evidence of heart disease. These studies are not definitive since the women were not randomly assigned to treatment. Also, women who participated in these studies were healthier, which may account for the lower incidence of heart attacks and strokes.

These new developments leave women and their doctors in a difficult place. HRT can be effective for decreasing the bone thinning of osteoporosis and for reducing menopausal hot flashes and vaginal dryness. However, HRT carries risks too. Any woman, with or without established heart disease, who is considering HRT should talk with her doctor about the benefits and risks. Use the information below to help you and your doctor make the right choice for you.

Known and Potential Benefits of HRT

- HRT raises "good" HDL cholesterol and lowers "bad" LDL cholesterol. Skin patches may not have these benefits.
- The long-term Nurses' Health Study found that healthy women who took HRT had a lower risk of heart disease and death from most major diseases (except breast cancer).
- HRT keeps arteries flexible and increases blood flow, which makes them more able to respond to exercise and physical stress.
- HRT can help relieve menopausal symptoms such as hot flashes and help prevent bone loss.

Known and Potential Risks of HRT

- HRT does not reduce the risk of heart attack or dying from CHD in women who have heart disease.
- HRT using estrogen alone increases the risk of endometrial and uterine cancers. Combining estrogen and progestin helps reduce the risk of endometrial cancer associated with estrogen.
- HRT increases the risk of gallbladder disease. Skin patches may not.
- It's unknown whether HRT increases breast cancer risk. Some studies show that it does; others show it does not.
- HRT raises triglyceride levels and possibly heart disease risk.
- Taking HRT when immobilized increases the risk for developing blood clots.
- Any woman who has the following conditions should be cautious about taking HRT.
  - Liver disease (active or chronic)
  - History of breast or uterine cancer, or a family history of breast cancer
  - Gallbladder disease
  - History of blood clots, especially in the veins of the legs or lungs
  - CHD
  - Obesity
  - Diabetes
  - High blood pressure
  - History of stroke

Reducing Your Risk

If you're a woman with CHD or concerned about CHD, here's how you can reduce your risk:

Identify your risk factors. Work closely with your doctor to determine exactly what your heart disease risk factors are.

Reduce your risk factors. Lower your risk by making healthy lifestyle changes. Eat a low-fat, low-cholesterol diet. Lose excess weight. Lower your high cholesterol and your high blood pressure. Quit smoking and limit alcohol to no more than one drink per day. See chapter 9 for more information on heart-healthy lifestyle changes.

Talk with your doctor about HRT. Carefully weigh the risks and benefits of taking HRT, especially if you have established heart disease.

Know women's warning signs of heart attack. Too often, women don't recognize when they're having a heart attack. Women often have subtler symptoms. Recognizing heart attack symptoms can save your life.

Respond to warning signs. Don't wait if you think you may be having a heart attack. Call for emergency medical help (911 or other number) immediately. (See chapter 4 for more advice about responding to a heart attack.)

Less Typical Heart Attack/Heart Disease Symptoms Often Experienced by Women

- Chronic breathlessness or waking at night with difficulty breathing
- Overwhelming, chronic fatigue
- Unexplained dizziness or blackouts
- Swelling, especially in the ankles and/or lower legs
- Rapid heartbeats
- Nausea or gastric upset

6

Getting a Diagnosis

Doctors today have a number of tests available to diagnose heart disease. The sooner your CHD is diagnosed, the sooner you can begin treatment to help prevent further atherosclerotic buildup (or in some cases, even reverse it) and help prevent a potentially deadly heart attack.

There is no single test for CHD. Diagnosing heart disease can be quite complicated because sometimes more than one type of heart disease occurs in the same person at the same time. Additionally, you may have other health problems that make it more difficult to determine exactly what's going on. To evaluate your heart health, your doctor has to be a bit of a detective. He or she will use a number of clues from a variety of sources to make a diagnosis. Your diagnosis will be based on:

- Your medical history/interview
- A physical examination
- Diagnostic tests

Your Medical History/Interview

The first thing your doctor will likely do is review your medical history and conduct a medical interview. Your medical history will include a number of questions about illnesses, surgeries, etc., that you or close family members have had. Providing complete and thorough information will help your doctor get a more accurate picture of your health. During the interview, your doctor will review your medical history with you and ask you a number of questions about your current state of health, including any symptoms you may be having. You should be prepared to answer questions such as:

- Have you or anyone in your family had a heart attack, stroke, or circulatory problem?
- What medications do you take?
- Have you ever had an abnormal electrocardiogram or exercise stress test?
- Have you ever taken heart medications or cholesterol-lowering medications?
- Describe your symptoms. When do these symptoms occur?
- What makes these symptoms better or worse?

Physical Examination

Once your doctor has thoroughly interviewed you about your medical history and your symptoms, he or she will conduct a physical exam. By listening, feeling and observing specific areas of your body, your doctor can get clues about what's going on. This includes checking your vital signs—pulse, blood pressure, breath rate. If you have no CHD symptoms, your doctor may detect signs of poor circulation elsewhere in your body. Using a stethoscope, he or she will listen to your heart for irregular sounds and examine your neck, abdomen, and elsewhere for evidence of "bruits" or rough sounds produced by turbulent blood flow through narrowed arteries. Your doctor will also listen to your lungs, looking for signs of extra fluid buildup.

By carefully observing the veins in the neck while you're in various positions, the doctor can detect elevated pressures on the right side of the heart. He or she will also look for skin that is cool and pale or bluish (*cyanotic*), a sign of vascular disease. Since severe atherosclerosis in the legs can cause hair loss and thickening of the toenails, the doctor should carefully examine your feet and legs. The doctor will look for evidence of swelling (*edema*), especially in your feet, ankles, and legs.

Diagnostic Tests

The diagnostic tests your doctor uses will depend on your symptoms, your medical history, your risk factors, and the results of your physical exam. The specific diagnostic tests selected will be tailored for you. If your history, your symptoms, and your physical examination don't indicate problems, your doctor will likely only order a few tests. Regardless of whether or not you have CHD symptoms, you'll probably need more than one diagnostic test because different tests provide the doctor with different information. Fortunately, many of the tests for CHD are *non-invasive*—they're done outside the body and are painless.

Common Diagnostic Tests for CHD

- Blood tests (lipid profile, blood count, chemistries)
- Electrocardiography (ECG)
- Chest X-ray
- Nuclear scanning and stress testing
- Catheterization and angiography
- Advanced imaging technology (CT, EBT, EBA, PET, MRI)

Electrocardiography (ECG)

One of the most common tests for heart disease, *electrocardiography (ECG)* records the electrical activity of the heart. (ECGs are also called EKGs.) Your doctor will likely order an ECG if you have CHD symptoms such as chest pain, shortness of breath, palpitations (rapid fluttering of the heart), or fainting. Some doctors like to do an ECG on anyone over age 40 during routine examinations.

The ECG is a painless, non-invasive test that takes less than 10 minutes. The doctor, nurse, or technician attaches twelve electrodes at various points on your body. Then you sit or lie quietly while the machine records the electrical activity of your heart. The results are recorded as "waves" displayed on a monitor or printed on a paper.

The ECG provides valuable information about your heart's rate, rhythm, whether you've previously had a heart attack, or have structural abnormalities. However, like most tests, it's not without limitations. A normal ECG doesn't rule out CHD. In fact, you may have a totally normal resting ECG and have a 90 percent narrowing of a major coronary artery. Unfortunately, ECG changes often don't occur until atherosclerosis is very severe or after structural damage has occurred.

Likewise, an abnormal ECG doesn't mean you definitely have CHD, particularly if you don't have CHD symptoms or CHD risk factors. ECG abnormalities can be caused by non-heart problems such as blood/tissue salt (electrolyte) abnormalities, lung disease, and some types of medication.

Exercise Stress Test

The *exercise stress test* is a recording of your heart's electrical activity under stress. It's also referred to as a stress ECG or a treadmill test. It's usually done while you're walking on a treadmill or pedaling a stationary bike. Because the stress test produces higher heart rates than the resting ECG (EKG), it's better able to detect problems such as poor circulation and insufficient blood and oxygen supply in the coronary arteries. The test is an excellent measure of how your heart muscle functions. The exercise test can also detect exercise-related heart rhythm disturbances and abnormalities in blood pressure response. If you've had a heart attack or you're already being treated for heart problems with medications, your doctor may order periodic stress ECG tests to check on the severity of the coronary artery obstruction and to monitor your progress. The test also can be used to design an exercise program that strengthens your heart.

If your doctor orders an exercise stress test for you:

- Plan for about an hour. You'll be asked to walk or pedal for 5 to 15 minutes. The rest of the time you'll be monitored at rest.

- Eat only a light breakfast or lunch before taking the test. Allow at least two hours between your meal and your exercise stress test.

- Take your medications as usual, unless directed otherwise. Some people need to stop taking their medications a day or two before the test, but your doctor will tell you if that's necessary. (Some tests are designed to detect a problem and medications are withheld. Other tests are to see how well the person is protected with medications.)

- Wear comfortable clothing and walking shoes.
- Let the doctor, nurse, or technician know immediately if you feel chest discomfort or shortness of breath during the test.

For most people, undergoing an exercise stress test is perfectly safe. Since the test stresses the heart, there is a very small risk of suffering a heart attack or serious rhythm disturbance, but the risk is very slight. Your doctor, nurses, and the technicians on hand are trained to handle any type of heart emergency that might occur.

The exercise stress test isn't for everyone. Some people cannot walk on a treadmill. Some have uninterpretable results that require a different type of stress test. An exercise stress test is *not* for you if you have:

- Chest pain (angina) at rest
- Potentially life-threatening heart rhythm problems (arrhythmias)
- Infection, inflammation, or swelling of the heart sac (pericarditis), heart muscle (myocarditis), or heart valves (endocarditis)
- Tear on the inner lining of the aorta (aortic dissection)
- Blood clots in the lungs (pulmonary infarct or embolus)
- Other serious or acute illness

The exercise stress test is a fairly reliable test for detecting severe coronary blockages of the main artery or blockages of all three major coronary vessels (at least 50 percent narrowed). However, it's not perfect. It will detect obstructive CHD in about 67 percent of those with the disease in one of the three major arteries. When the test is negative, it does not give any information about the presence or absence of plaque. Your doctor will interpret the results of your exercise test in concert with your symptoms, your medical history, your risk factors, and other test results.

Ambulatory ECG (Holter Monitoring)

A variation on the exercise stress test, an *ambulatory ECG* (also called *Holter monitoring* for its inventor) monitors the heart during everyday activities. This test can help detect heart problems that seem to come and go. Holter monitoring involves electrodes attached to the chest and a portable recording device (the size of a Walkman) that records the heart's electrical activity. It can detect abnormal heart rhythms and changes related to lack of blood flow. You keep the device on for a 24-hour period, even when you're sleeping. The doctor will also likely ask you to maintain a symptom diary to correlate different types of activity with ECG results.

Chest X-ray

Your doctor may order a chest X-ray to look at the size and shape of your heart and major blood vessels. A chest X-ray also lets the doctor examine your lungs, which may suggest heart problems. If your heart isn't pumping strongly enough, for instance, fluid may leak into the air sacs of the lungs (*pulmonary edema*).

A chest X-ray is quick and painless. You'll be asked to remove your clothing and jewelry from the waist up and put on a hospital gown. You'll stand against a plate that holds the X-ray film with your arms held up or out to the sides. You'll be asked to take a breath and hold it, which helps the heart and lungs show up on the X-ray.

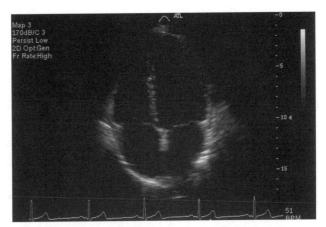

During an echocardiogram, sound waves produce an image of the beating heart. The test measures heart function and can also detect narrowing of arteries when coupled with stress testing.

Having a chest X-ray with today's low-dose machines is quite safe. However, if you're pregnant, be sure to tell your doctor before having a chest X-ray. Risk to the baby is low, but special precautions should be taken to protect the baby from exposure. A chest X-ray during pregnancy is done only when absolutely necessary.

Echocardiography

A technology that's been around for at least 40 years, *echocardiography* uses high-pitched sound waves (*ultrasound*) sent out to your heart to reflect back a "picture" of your heart. Ultrasound uses the same principles that bats or submarines use to navigate. Echocardiography is a non-invasive procedure that provides precise information about your heart's function, its valves, and adjacent structures.

One type of ultrasound, the Doppler, provides heart sounds and displays an image of the blood flowing between different chambers of the heart. A color map (color Doppler) and other precise measurements can be made with the Doppler ultrasound to assess the severity of narrowing in a heart valve. It can also non-invasively measure the pressure inside the lungs.

Sometimes doctors use echocardiography to picture the heart under stress (a *stress echocardiogram*). You might be asked to walk on a treadmill or take a medication (dobutamine) that causes the heart to beat faster and stronger for a few minutes. This enables doctors to compare ultrasound images of the heart both at rest and under stress. A stress echocardiogram is slightly less accurate than nuclear scanning for detecting obstructive narrowing, but more accurate than an ECG stress test.

Your echocardiogram is usually done in the cardiologist's office or laboratory (or in the hospital if you're hospitalized). You don't have to do anything special before having the test. You'll be asked to remove your clothing from the waist up and put on a hospital gown or drape. You'll lie down on your back or left side. After having a special gel applied to your chest (the gel improves the transmission of ultrasound waves), the doctor, nurse, or lab technician will move an instrument (a *transducer*) over your chest. The transducer is attached to a monitoring screen and other components. The examination is painless and will take 15 to 30 minutes. There is no known risk to using ultrasound.

Certain conditions make it difficult to get a clear ultrasound image. Such conditions include:

- having lung disease (such as emphysema)
- being very overweight or underweight
- having spinal or chest wall abnormalities
- having very large breasts or breast implants

- having had chest or heart surgery or a chest injury
- if you're on a ventilator

A specialized type of echocardiogram is the *transesophageal echocardiogram* (TEE). It magnifies the heart's structures (including the valves) and can detect blood clots that are hiding in the left atrium. These hidden clots can travel and may cause a stroke. TEE is also used in some people during open-heart surgery to check the valves and heart muscle function. Unlike other forms of echocardiography, TEE is somewhat invasive. The test takes approximately 20 minutes and is usually done on an outpatient basis. The throat is numbed with a local anesthesia and a tube is passed to the esophagus, which lies directly behind the heart. The tube contains a tiny ultrasound crystal that reflects back the ultra-sound image.

Nuclear Scanning

Nuclear scans can determine whether or not the heart is receiving enough blood flow under stress. Depending on the type of scan selected, nuclear scanning can tell the doctor about the size of the chambers of the heart, how the ventricles are pumping blood, and blood flow to the heart muscle and lungs. Additionally, the doctor may order nuclear scans to monitor the effectiveness of medication or to see how much improvement there is in blood flow to the heart following angioplasty or bypass surgery.

This imaging technology involves a tiny amount of radio-active material injected into the bloodstream. The material gives off miniscule amounts of energy (radiation) that can be detected by specialized cameras. Many people are alarmed by the idea of injecting radioactive material into their bodies. However, the amount of radiation you'll be exposed to is very small and is safe. The benefits of the tests outweigh the small risk. However, if you're pregnant or possibly pregnant, you should avoid these tests.

It's very rare to have adverse reactions to isotopes. Some people who receive drugs used to simulate the stress of exercise, develop headache, a warm sensation, chest discomfort, or shortness of breath. These symptoms usually go away in a short time. If needed, they can be reversed with medication.

There are several types of nuclear scans. Each one uses a different radioactive material, or *isotope*. The isotopes have different properties, which allows each one to detect different heart problems.

When Are Nuclear Scans Performed?

Nuclear scans are taken at rest and then again right after exercising—walking on a treadmill or bicycling. It generally takes 15 to 20 minutes to take the pictures each time. Some doctors like to take the resting scan first and then immediately follow with the stress test and post-stress scan. Others prefer to conduct the stress test and then do the resting scan four hours later.

The nuclear scans compare the heart under stress and at rest. Unfortunately, a blockage must be pretty severe—at least 50 percent blocked—before it can be detected with nuclear scanning. They can detect narrowing in 88 to 90 percent of people with these serious blockages. A negative test can rule out severe obstructions in most people, but it doesn't eliminate the possibility of severe plaque in the arteries.

Single Photon Emission Computed Tomography (SPECT)

One of the most widely used nuclear scans is *single photon emission computed tomography (SPECT)*. It involves injecting a radioactive tracer and then taking images of the chest area. Once the images are captured, a sophisticated computer "slices" the images, giving precise pictures that enable the doctor to visualize blood flow problems both at rest and during exercise. This technology enables the doctor to assess blood flow to the heart muscle to see how well the heart muscle is functioning in the different regions of the heart. This technology is able to indirectly locate and determine the significance of blood flow blockages.

Multigated Acquisition (MUGA)

The *multigated acquisition (MUGA)*, may be used to assess heart muscle function at rest and under stress. MUGA allows doctors to see areas of the heart that have been damaged by previous heart attack or that are deprived of circulation.

Your doctor may ask you to stop taking your heart medication a day or two before your test. Don't stop taking your heart medication unless instructed by your doctor. To avoid nausea, your doctor may also ask you not to eat or drink for several hours before the scan. In most cases, nuclear tests can be performed in the doctor's office. If you're hospitalized, you'll be evaluated at the hospital.

Advanced Imaging Techniques

Recent developments in technology have allowed for even more sophisticated imaging of the heart and may enable doctors to diagnose CHD before a person has symptoms.

Standard Cardiac Computed Tomography (CT)

X-ray computed tomography (also known as a CT or CAT scan) produces cross-sectional images of the chest, including the heart, the lungs, and major blood vessels. It's especially helpful in evaluating diseases of the large blood vessels, masses or tumors in the heart, and diseases of the heart sac. It's also helpful in diagnosing blood clots on the lung or tears of the aorta.

The images are produced by passing an X-ray beam through the body. Unlike a regular X-ray machine, the CT X-ray machine is rapidly rotated around the body. This allows images to be captured from various angles. A computer then combines the images and produces a detailed cross section of the body. Though there is a small amount of exposure to radiation, all CT scans are painless and involve little risk.

Electron Beam Tomography (EBT) or Electron Beam Computed Tomography (EBCT)

Also called "ultra-fast CT" or EBCT, EBT is a newer, specialized type of CT scan. In many instances, it can diagnose atherosclerosis *before* the blockages become too severe, which can be life saving. EBT is to heart disease what the mammogram is to breast cancer—early detection.

EBT detects the presence of calcium in blood vessels. Calcium itself does not cause heart attack, but its presence is an

Electron Beam Tomography of Coronary Arteries

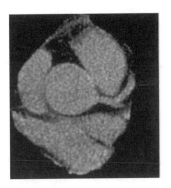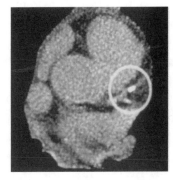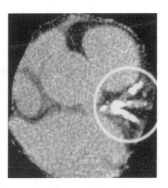

EBT photographs the heart between beats and measures calcium in plaque deposits attached to artery walls. The higher the EBT calcium score, the greater the risk of heart attack. An example of a normal heart, without calcification, is shown on the left. Moderate and severe calcification are demonstrated in the midle and right.

important indicator of CHD and potentially in predicting heart attack risk. In the plaque building of atherosclerosis, the blood vessel walls are continually being injured and the body is constantly attempting to heal the injuries. As the body tries to repair the damaged area, calcium is deposited in the injured area. On routine X-rays, this hard calcium shows up only at a very late stage. With EBT, calcium deposits can be detected and measured at a very early stage. The amount of calcium detected by EBT is related to the amount of underlying coronary athero-sclerosis. Having a high EBT calcium score can predict the risk for future cardiac events like heart attacks. The reliability of prediction by EBT was recently confirmed by a landmark study conducted by the Mayo Clinic. Having a negative EBT calcium score implies a low risk for plaques that may block coronary arteries and a lower risk for heart attacks.

Studies have demonstrated that EBT calcium scores are more accurate than traditional risk factors (smoking, diabetes, high blood pressure, high cholesterol) for determining a person's risk for heart disease and subsequent heart attacks. When the researchers combined EBT scores with risk factors, they were able to predict risk even more accurately.

EBT involves taking high-resolution X-rays of the heart. A computer reconstructs the many images and displays the combined image on a screen. Your doctor can examine the EBT calcium in the plaque of the three major coronary arteries feeding the heart. EBT is fast and painless. No intravenous or X-ray dyes are used. Results are available immediately, allowing further diagnostic procedures or prevention strategies to be started immediately.

People who are likely candidates for EBT include:

- Men age 35+ and women age 45+
- Past or present smokers
- People who have a sedentary lifestyle
- People who have a stressful lifestyle
- Those with diabetes
- People with high blood pressure
- Those with high LDL cholesterol or low HDL cholesterol
- People who are overweight
- Those who suffer from other vascular disease (such as carotid artery narrowing)

Note: Women who are pregnant should wait until after delivery before having the test.

Jim is an active, 62-year-old physician. He's never smoked and has mild high blood pressure. His "bad" LDL cholesterol is slightly elevated and he has low "good" HDL cholesterol. He has diabetes, but he controls his blood sugar with diabetic pills. Last year, his stress test was normal and he refused cholesterol medications. Jim's father died at 57 of a heart attack, but Jim wasn't really concerned about his own heart health.

One day a fellow physician saw Jim in the hospital corridor and recommended he get an EBT. He agreed and the test showed that Jim's calcium score was higher than 90 percent of men his age—not a good sign. Reluctantly, Jim agreed to a nuclear stress test. His EKG response looked normal, but the nuclear pictures showed some abnormality. Jim was still hesitant to believe that anything was really wrong. At his wife's insistence, Jim agreed to undergo cardiac catheterization. It showed he had a critical 90 percent narrowing of the left main coronary artery. If Jim had waited, his first coronary event would have been sudden death.

Fortunately, Jim immediately went in for bypass surgery. He was discharged in five days and was back at work within six weeks. He has changed his lifestyle. He has increased his exercise program and has started following a heart-healthy diet. He's also taking diabetic, blood pressure, and cholesterol medications.

Although EBT has the potential to detect CHD earlier than many other tests, it has limitations. Older people—men over 65 and women over 75—all have some coronary calcification. In this older age group, EBT can't distinguish between normal, age-related calcium and calcium that's related to CHD. While EBT isn't a substitute for clinically indicated cardiac catheterization, studies continue to verify that it can be an effective weapon in the early detection of CHD. Some critics suggest that the type of plaque deposits that EBT is most likely to detect may not be the type likely to cause heart attack. Some researchers don't believe the measurement of coronary calcium is helpful in people who have already had a heart attack or have undergone coronary bypass surgery or coronary angioplasty. Other scientists believe EBT may be a useful tool to follow the removal of plaque and can be a tool for cholesterol-lowering therapy.

Bob is a 42-year-old runner and father of three young children. He was concerned because his father, who was a heavy smoker, had died at age 45 from a heart attack. Bob had never smoked, wasn't diabetic, and had normal blood pressure. His bad LDL cholesterol was slightly elevated and his good HDL cholesterol was high, probably the result of all of Bob's exercising. However, because of his positive family history for heart disease and his LDL cholesterol level, his internist wanted him to start a cholesterol medicine (statin). Bob resisted, fearing that he'd end up taking medication for the rest of his life. Instead, he took an EBT test, which showed he had absolutely no evidence of any plaque. His doctor advised him to continue his heart-healthy lifestyle without medications. They'd followup in a couple of years (or immediately if any symptoms occurred).

Electron Beam Angiography (EBA)

This is a non-invasive angiogram of the arteries that feed the heart. EBA requires an EBT machine and an intravenous injection of X-ray dye. It does not involve inserting catheters and takes only about 30 minutes. Previously, EBA was used only to evaluate those who'd undergone coronary artery bypass graft surgery (CABG) to see whether the bypasses were still functioning. Because it also provides the calcium score, EBA is now being used in some people to assess the coronary arteries and can help avoid some unnecessary procedures.

Cardiac Positron-Emission Tomography (PET)

This technology is used to measure blood flow and metabolism in the heart. Although it's fairly new in cardiac imaging and more expensive than some other imaging technologies, PET has the advantage of letting doctors see how the heart uses energy, which may give them new information about heart metabolism and function. This technology is a very accurate, non-invasive way to detect CHD. It can also identify injured heart tissue. Studies suggest PET may play an important role in diagnosing patients, in identifying the extent of CHD, and in developing a treatment strategy.

PET involves imaging radionuclide tracers (small amounts of radiation) in the bloodstream and creating a computerized image. The widespread use of PET has been limited, in part because it's expensive.

Magnetic Resonance Imaging (MRI)

Formally called nuclear magnetic resonance (NMR) imaging, MRI relies on powerful magnets and radio waves to look inside the body and create images of the structures within. MRI can give your doctor a look at your heart muscle, help identify if your heart has suffered any damage from a previous heart attack, and evaluate diseases of the larger blood vessels. New research suggests MRI can detect plaque buildup in a carotid artery that is likely to rupture. Cardiac MRI may also prove to be a tool to do non-invasive arteriography, especially for those who can't tolerate X-ray dye (such as those with kidney disease).

MRI doesn't use ionizing radiation like standard X-rays or CT scans. There are no known risks from using MRI. It produces clear, high-resolution, three-dimensional images of the heart's chambers and large vessels without having to use contrast agents. In addition, adjacent bone and air doesn't interfere with the images. However, because MRI depends on magnetic forces, if you have a pacemaker or other metal in the body, you can't undergo the test.

There are also newer types of MRI technology. One of them is *fast cine MRI*. Using a new form of high-speed MRI, the machine is able to view the wall of the heart as it beats and picture the heart as it expands and contracts, nearly as it's happening. Fast cine MRI can be combined with the drug dobutamine to produce pictures of the heart under stress. Dobutamine, which acts like adrenaline, mimics the stress of exercise and causes a reduction in the blood supplied to the heart. Doctors using the high-speed MRI can evaluate the ability of the left ventricular wall to move during stress and get a clear, three-dimensional image of the heart in motion. The new test takes about 35 minutes to perform. According to researchers at Wake Forest University School of Medicine who are studying this newer MRI, the test has proved to be an accurate predictor of CHD. Among those who tested negative with the fast cine MRI, 97 percent were event-free within one year of testing.

Cardiac Catheterization and Angiography

Also called coronary angiography, arteriography, or angiocardiography, this invasive diagnostic technique can show blood flow problems and blockages in the coronary arteries. It can measure blood pressure in the heart, determine how much oxygen is in the blood, and provide information about the structure and function of the heart muscle, heart valves, and arteries. Because techniques have become so refined, you may be able to have a therapeutic procedure (angioplasty or stenting) during this diagnostic procedure. (See chapter 8 for more information on angioplasty and stenting.)

During cardiac catheterization and angiography, a long, sterile, flexible tube called a *catheter* is threaded through an artery in the leg or arm into the heart. Then a liquid contrast material is injected into the tube. The contrast material allows the heart and blood vessels to show up on an X-ray videotape called an *angiogram* or *arteriogram.*

Your doctor may order cardiac catheterization and angiography as a diagnostic tool if:

- He or she suspects you have significant CHD
- You'll be undergoing heart surgery such as bypass surgery
- You have heart valve problems, including valve narrowing (stenosis), or blood backflow through an abnormal valve (insufficiency)

- He or she suspects you have heart muscle damage (cardiomyopathy)

Cardiac catheterization and angiography is done in a special *catheterization laboratory* (*cath lab*) in a hospital.

Before the Cardiac Catherization:

- Don't eat or drink anything after midnight the night before the procedure (except small amounts of water for taking medication). If catheterization is scheduled for the afternoon, your doctor may allow you to have clear liquids for breakfast.
- Empty your bladder before the exam.
- Leave jewelry at home.
- Inform your doctor if you're allergic to X-ray dye. Most hospitals use the newer X-ray dyes, which decrease (but do not totally eliminate) allergic reactions. Doctors pre-treat those who have dye allergies with antihistamines and corticosteroids to reduce the likelihood of an allergic reaction.
- If you're pregnant, be sure to let your doctor know.

The area on your leg or arm where the catheter will be inserted will be cleaned and shaved. An intravenous line will be inserted into your arm to deliver fluids and medications. Then you'll be taken to the cath lab and placed on a flat table under an X-ray machine. The nurses will attach electrocardiogram electrodes to your arms and legs and you'll be given medication to help you relax. A blood pressure cuff will be put on your arm, and a *pulse oximeter* (a non-invasive, clothespin-like monitor for blood oxygen content) will be placed on your finger.

You likely won't be totally asleep during the procedure, but you may doze. The cardiologist and other members of your cath team will likely explain what's being done throughout the process and let you know what sensations to expect. The doctor numbs the insertion site, usually the area over the femoral artery located in the groin. An artery at the wrist or at the inside elbow may be used, especially if leg arteries have severe blockages. The cardiologist inserts a needle into the vessel, and then threads a thin guide wire through the needle. After withdrawing the needle, the doctor inserts a flexible tube called a *sheath* into the blood vessel over the guide wire. The sheath has a one-way valve in it that allows the catheter to be inserted, but keeps blood from leaking out.

In rare cases, an incision is made to access the artery. This technique known as a *cutdown*, was more common in the past. It takes a little longer and requires stitches to repair the incision.

By watching the X-ray video carefully to monitor the progress, the doctor advances the catheter through the blood vessels to your heart. During the procedure, the cardiologist may insert several catheters via the same entry site into various parts of your heart. You don't feel the catheter when it's inside. Once in the heart, the catheter(s) can perform functions such as measuring the pressure in the chambers, taking blood samples, and injecting X-ray dye (also called contrast) for an angiogram (pictures of arteries).

When contrast material is injected into the main pumping chamber of the heart or into the main artery, you'll feel a hot sensation that lasts for 5 to 20 seconds. It's important to remain very still so that the X-ray images will be clear. You may also feel your heart "skip beats." Occasionally, you may feel nauseated or hot all over during the procedure, which usually passes after a minute or so. These are all normal sensations and shouldn't alarm you. However, let the doctor know when you experience these feelings or if you feel any chest pain.

After Cardiac Catheterization

After all the tests and procedures are completed, the catheter(s) will be removed. The insertion site will be compressed or the cardiologist will insert a closure device. About 20 minutes of compression allows the body to make its own blood clot to seal the opening. A specialized pressure dressing may then be applied to the wound to help prevent bleeding. After the catheterization, you'll be required to lie flat on your back for 6 to 8 hours with your leg extended. Arm procedures don't require prolonged bedrest. During this time, the cath nurse will monitor your vital signs and keep an eye on the catheter insertion site to make sure it's not bleeding. He or she will also monitor the pulse, color, and temperature of the arm or leg used for the procedure. Let the nurse know if you notice any swelling, bleeding, or pain where the catheter was placed. If your doctor used a closure device (stitches, plugs, or a type of sealer) on the insertion site, the required bed rest time is much shorter—as little as an hour. Once you've recovered sufficiently, the doctor will release you to go home.

Before leaving the clinic or hospital, you may wish to talk to your physician about the following:

- Ask about results. You can usually talk with your doctor about your condition right after the procedure.

Your doctor will likely come into the recovery room and talk with you about your results. He or she will also let your family know the results right after the procedure.

- Ask the doctor when you can resume eating and drinking.
- Have someone available to drive you home. You shouldn't drive for at least 24 hours following the procedure.
- Avoid strenuous activity for at least 48 hours after the procedure.
- Call the doctor's office immediately if the catheter insertion site becomes swollen, red, painful, or oozes blood, or if the limb becomes painful, cold and pale, or has a weak or absent pulse.
- Return to the doctor's office for follow-up within 5 to 7 days.

Risks of Cardiac Catheterization

While cardiac catheterization and angiography can provide your doctor with valuable information about your heart's health, it's not without risk. In most cases, the procedure is safe. However, serious complications are possible such as stroke or heart attack, abnormal heartbeat (arrhythmia), puncture of a blood vessel or the heart muscle, bleeding, blood clotting or infection at the site of insertion, a blocked blood vessel in the arm or leg where the catheter was inserted, or an allergic reaction to the X-ray dye. Keep in mind that serious complications are rare. They usually occur in people who are critically ill or when catheterization is done under emergency conditions.

You're at greater risk for serious complications if you have chronic illnesses such as kidney failure, insulin-dependent diabetes, severe lung disease, severely decreased heart function, or if you're older than 80 years. If you have kidney problems, you're at greater risk for dye-related kidney complications. Your cath team will need to take special precautions to minimize your risk and avoid problems.

Coping After a Diagnosis of CHD

If your diagnostic tests indicate that you have CHD, don't forget that there can be an emotional impact on you. It's easy to think of CHD as a purely physical disease. However, the diagnosis of heart disease is bound to affect you emotionally. In fact, depression is a very common response to the diagnosis of CHD or following a heart attack or heart surgery. It's often triggered by feelings of loss—perhaps loss of the way your body once was or loss of the old, familiar lifestyle. Or it may be triggered by fears—of dying, of having another heart attack, or of feeling vulnerable and frail.

If you find yourself unable to sleep, tearful, or having feelings of hopelessness and despair, talk with your doctor. He or she can provide treatment for your symptoms of depression.

Here are some other strategies for dealing with depression, anxiety, or fears about your heart disease:

Avoid denial. Don't block out your physical problem hoping it will "just go away."

Cry. Allow yourself to feel your feelings deeply. Acknowledge that having heart disease is an emotionally painful condition.

Avoid withdrawal. Don't wall yourself off from others. Stay involved with family, friends, and colleagues.

Talk to others. Call friends or close family members and talk about how you feel. Set yourself a goal to talk to someone for at least a few minutes every day.

Join a group. There are support groups for cardiac patients. Ask your doctor for a referral.

Get out. You may have to force yourself to go out at first, but do it. Accept every invitation.

Keep a journal. Just writing down how you feel can help. When you've finished writing down all your negative feelings, start a new page with the heading "Things I'm Doing for Myself Today."

7

Medications for Coronary Heart Disease

Now that your doctor has confirmed that you have coronary heart disease, undoubtedly your next question is "What do I do about it?" Your treatment will depend on the severity of your CHD and your general health. CHD treatment aims to prevent or reverse significant artery narrowing and make sure your heart gets enough oxygen to prevent it from becoming damaged and having a heart attack. Medications can help, especially if you have chest pain or if you have high blood pressure or high blood cholesterol.

A number of medications have proven effective in treating CHD and its risk factors. For many people, drug therapy can help prevent a heart attack or stroke. It can help prevent complications and slow the progression of atherosclerosis. Unlike surgical options, heart medications aren't invasive. They're also less expensive.

All drugs, however, have *side effects*. These are unwanted or undesirable effects. Some of these are minor; others are more serious. For anyone taking medication, the benefits of the medication must be weighed against the risks. That's why it's important that you only take heart medication under the direction and close supervision of your doctor.

Keep a current list of all your medications, including the names, dosages, and when and how you take them. Share this list with your doctor and your pharmacist to ensure you aren't taking medications that may dangerously interact. Let your doctor know about any medications that have caused you problems in the past such as rashes, dizziness, indigestion, or poor appetite.

Commonly Used CHD Medications

A number of medications are used to prevent and/or treat CHD. Your doctor may prescribe one or a combination of medications for you, depending on the nature of your CHD and other health problems. Medications for CHD include:

- Anti-anginal medications
  - Nitrates
  - Beta-blockers
  - Calcium channel blockers

- Blood thinners
  - Antiplatelet agents
  - Anticoagulants
  - Thrombolytics

- Cholesterol-lowering medications
  - Statins
  - Fibrates
  - Resins
  - Nicotinic acid

- Medications to lower blood pressure
  - ACEs and ARBs
  - Diuretics
  - Beta-blockers
  - Calcium channel blockers
  - Alpha-blockers
  - Nerve inhibitors
  - Vasodilators

Anti-anginal Medications

Nitrates

Often prescribed to relieve angina, *nitrates*—usually nitro-glycerine—widen the coronary arteries. This increases blood flow to the heart. They also dilate the veins, which slows the return of blood to the heart and makes the heart work less.

If you have severe angina, your doctor may prescribe nitro-glycerine (NTG) tablets or spray that you put under your tongue. It works very fast to relieve pain. If you need daily doses of nitrate medication, your doctor may prescribe it in a capsule or as a cream or patch that's placed on the skin. Even if you take long-acting preparations (pills or patches) you may still need to take nitrate tablets or spray, as needed, if break-through pain occurs. Intravenous NTG is available for patients who are hospitalized.

The most problematic side effect of nitrate medication is a sudden drop in blood pressure when you stand from sitting or lying down (*orthostatic hypotension*). If your systolic blood pressure is below 90 mmHg, nitroglycerine probably isn't a good choice. The medication can also cause flushing, headache, dizziness, and rapid heartbeat (*tachycardia*). Some side effects such as headache usually lessen after taking the medication for several days. In rare cases, topical nitrates can cause a skin rash. Alcohol may worsen side effects.

Never take nitroglycerine if you've been taking Viagra (sildenafil). It can cause a life-threatening drop in blood pressure. If you've been taking Viagra and you're having chest pain—even severe chest pain—*don't* take nitroglycerine. Instead, go to the hospital immediately.

All forms of nitrates have a limited shelf life. Nitrates that are too old simply won't work. Talk with your pharmacist about how long your nitrates will be effective and how to store them to keep them at their peak.

Commonly prescribed nitrates: nitroglycerine (*NTG, Nitro-Bid, Nitrostat, Nitrogard*). Longer-acting preparations such as isosorbide mononitrate or dinitrate (*ISMO, Monoket, Imdur, Sorbitrate, Isordil*).

Beta-Blockers

Beta-blockers are another type of drug commonly prescribed for angina. Beta-blockers decrease heart rate, reduce the strength of the heart's contractions, and lower blood pressure. As a result, they decrease the heart's need for oxygen. When you drive your car at 50 miles per hour instead of 80 miles per hour, you use less gas. The same principle applies to the heart. The slower the heart rate, the less fuel or oxygen the heart needs. Beta-blockers can also help normalize some types of heart rhythm disturbances (abnormal beats). Additionally, this medication has been proven to decrease sudden death in people after a heart attack and to reduce the severity of a heart attack when given immediately.

Beta-blockers can also have a number of side effects. They may provoke wheezing and breathlessness in people with asthma. If you have coronary spasm, beta-blockers can worsen your angina. Abruptly stopping beta-blockers may cause an increase in heart rate and blood pressure. In some cases, beta-blockers worsen heart failure. However, long term, they've proven to improve symptoms and decrease mortality in people with heart failure. Other side effects include fatigue, dizziness, depression, diarrhea, skin rash, and sexual dysfunction.

Commonly prescribed beta-blockers: atenolol (*Tenormin*), metoprolol (*Lopressor, Toprol XL*), nadolol (*Corgard*), propranolol (*Inderal*), carvedilol (*Coreg*) in patients with heart failure.

Calcium Channel Blockers

As the name implies, *calcium channel blockers* block or inhibit the movement of calcium in the heart, nerves, and blood vessel walls. They reduce blood pressure and dilate coronary arteries, making them useful in treating angina (including the type caused by spasm). They also normalize some types of arrhythmias. People who aren't helped by or can't take nitro-glycerine or beta-blockers can often get relief using calcium channel blockers.

If you're taking calcium channel blockers, avoid drinking grapefruit juice at the time you take the medication. Grapefruit juice contains a component that interferes with the liver's ability to clear certain drugs such as nifedipine *(Adalat, Procardia)*, felodipine *(Plendil)* and nimodipine *(Nimotop)*. Drinking grapefruit juice and taking these drugs can allow toxic levels of the drugs to build up in the blood.

Commonly prescribed calcium channel blockers: diltiazem hydrochloride (*Cardizem, Dilacor, Cartia XT*), amlodipine (*Norvasc*), felodipine (*Plendil*), nimodipine (*Nimotop*), nifedipine (*Adalat, Procardia*), and verapamil (*Calan, Isoptin, Verelan, Covera*).

Blood Thinners

The body defends itself against bleeding to death by forming blood clots. However, blood's tendency to clot in the coronary arteries can also cause angina and heart attacks. There are two major ways that blood clots:

- Platelets, tiny cells circulating in the bloodstream, stick to damaged surfaces and to one another to form a so-called white clot (*white thrombus*).
- Specialized blood proteins are activated and form a gel-like red ball or red clot (*red thrombus*).

Blood thinners work to alter one or both of these blood-clotting mechanisms.

Antiplatelet Agents

These drugs reduce the blood's ability to clot by inhibiting the normal functioning of platelets. Aspirin is one of the best-known antiplatelet medications. It helps prevent blood clot formation on existing plaque, which reduces the risk of heart attacks. Over time, aspirin makes the blood more resistant to forming clots. Aspirin is usually prescribed to all patients with CHD unless they have an allergy or other problem. It's the first medication that's given in an emergency room during a heart attack. It's also used after coronary angioplasty and stenting to prevent blood clots and helps prolong the lifespan of bypasses created during coronary bypass surgery. (See chapter 8 for more information on these procedures.)

Thienopyridines—clopidogrel (*Plavix*) and ticlopidine (*Ticlid*)—are stronger than aspirin and are used with aspirin after coronary stenting to prevent a clot from forming on the stent. Typically these drugs have been prescribed for 1 month after having a stent placed. Recent studies show a significant benefit continuing clopidogrel for up to 9 months. Some patients may require them longer, especially if they had a coronary event despite taking aspirin. For people who receive intracoronary radiation for recurrent blockages, the prescription for these blood thinners is usually 12 months in addition to aspirin.

Clopidogrel is the drug of choice because of its low rate of side effects. Ticlopidine is only used if the person has an allergy to clopidogrel (rare) and taking this drug requires blood testing every two weeks to monitor for severe reductions in white blood cell count. This drug also causes a rash more frequently.

The most potent available antiplatelet drugs are intra-venous *glycoprotein llb/llla antagonists* including abciximab (*ReoPro*), eptifibatide (*Integrilin*), and tirofiban (*Aggrastat*). They are only given in the hospital to people who have unstable angina, heart attack, or during angioplasty and stenting. They can dramatically improve the treatment outcomes for people who have unstable angina and for higher-risk patients in cath labs.

Commonly prescribed antiplatelet agents: aspirin and clopidogrel (*Plavix*).

Anticoagulants

These blood-thinning drugs inhibit the specialized blood proteins that form the red blood clot (red thrombus). They are often given during and after a heart attack to prevent clots from forming. Your doctor may also prescribe an anticoagulant medication if you have atrial fibrillation (a type of irregular heartbeating) or an artificial heart valve. These drugs don't dissolve existing blood clots. They can, however, prevent new clots from forming or prevent existing clots from getting bigger. They can be administered both intravenously and by mouth.

The most common oral anticoagulant is warfarin (*Coumadin*), which interferes with blood clotting by blocking the body's use of vitamin K. The drug takes two to three days to start working and a similar amount of time to stop working. Dosage varies greatly from person to person. If you take warfarin, you'll need to have your blood checked regularly to ensure the dosage is right for you. If the dose is too little, the blood will be too thick and clotting may occur. If the dose is too much, the blood will be too thin and there's a risk of bleeding complications.

A number of drugs—antibiotics, steroids, diuretics, antidepressants, and pain relievers, among others—can interact with warfarin and cause serious complications. It's important to consult your doctor any time a new medication is prescribed for you. The drug can be used long-term for valve problems, some heart rhythm disturbances (atrial fibrillation), and for some people with CHD. Under close supervision, warfarin can be used in combination with aspirin.

Intravenous heparin is the classic intravenous anticoagulant used in hospitals. Newer agents called low molecular weight heparins have been developed (enoxaparin, dalteparin, tinzaparin) that are purer forms of heparin. They work better for some people. For instance, enoxaparin has proven to be superior to heparin for people with unstable angina and heart attack.

In rare cases, some people may be allergic to all heparin-based drugs. If you're one of these rare individuals, your cardiologist will prescribe an alternate medication when you're hospitalized.

Commonly prescribed oral anticoagulant: warfarin (*Coumadin*).

If you're taking any type of blood-thinning medication:

- Take the medication exactly as your doctor instructs
- Ask your doctor before taking other medications or supplements, even vitamins or over-the-counter medications
- Ask for any interactions with foods (Vitamin K in broccoli and spinach)
- Be sure to have blood tests regularly so your doctor can monitor how well your medications are working
- Tell your doctor about these (and any other medications you're taking) before you have surgery
- Watch for warning signs and let your doctor know right away if you have:
  - Pink or red urine
  - Red, black, or dark brown stools
  - Heavy menstrual bleeding (more than normal)
  - Bleeding gums

- Intense headache or stomach pain that doesn't go away
- Weakness, dizziness, fainting, or a general feeling of being unwell
- Bruises or blood blisters
- Pregnancy
- An accident of any kind (which could cause bleeding)

Thrombolytics

These clot-busting drugs are used to dissolve blood clots during a heart attack. They work by increasing the blood level and action of an enzyme (*plasmin*) that breaks up blood clots. While thrombolytics can't prevent a heart attack, they can help you survive one. To be effective, thrombolytics must be administered within the first few hours of a heart attack. They're most effective if they're given within the first hour.

The major risk with thrombolytics is bleeding, especially bleeding into the brain. This is relatively rare (up to 1.5 percent of cases) and occurs more frequently in women over the age of 70.

Commonly prescribed thrombolytics: tissue plasminogen activator or tPA (*Activase*), reteplase or rPA (*Retavase*), tenecteplase (*TNKASE*), and streptokinase (*Kabikinase, Streptase*).

Cholesterol-Lowering Medications

The newest guidelines from the National Institutes of Health's National Cholesterol Education Program say that the optimal level of LDL is less than 100 mg/dL. If you have CHD, one of your treatment goals will be to reduce your LDL cholesterol to 100 mg/dL or less. In addition to lifestyle changes, your doctor may prescribe cholesterol-lowering medications. All cholesterol-lowering medications are used with dietary therapy and need to be taken for at least a few years, sometimes for life.

A variety of drugs are available for lowering cholesterol. Some common types are *statins, resins, nicotinic acid*, and *fibrates*. Your doctor may prescribe a combination of drugs, especially if a single cholesterol-lowering medication doesn't adequately lower your cholesterol.

Statins

Statins are fast becoming the drugs of choice for reducing cholesterol. Statins enhance the body's ability to rid itself of cholesterol. They work directly on the liver to block a substance your body needs to manufacture cholesterol. The result is that cholesterol in the liver becomes depleted and cholesterol is removed from the circulating blood.

Statins are especially effective in reducing LDL cholesterol. Some studies indicate that statins can reduce LDL cholesterol by 30 to 40 percent, usually enough to bring cholesterol levels within safe limits. Statins may also help the body reabsorb cholesterol from plaques, slowly reversing atherosclerosis. Statins have been proven to reduce the risk of death from CHD, including the risk of a second heart attack.

Statins are easy to take, have few drug interactions, and few short-term side effects. Your doctor should also monitor your statin use with tests for liver function and muscle inflammation to ensure you're not having any problems with the drugs. A rare side effect is a serious muscle breakdown called rhabdomyolysis most notably described in patients taking a statin and fibrate (for high triglycerides) together. Warning signs of muscle damage would include: dark urine and muscle aches, weakness, fever, nausea, and vomiting. At the first sign of these problems, stop taking the medication immediately and contact your doctor. If caught early, problems from this uncommon side effect can be quickly and effectively treated. Statins also should not be used if you're pregnant or if you have chronic liver disease. In a few cases, people are allergic to statins and need to choose other cholesterol-lowering drugs.

Because the body makes more cholesterol at night, statins are usually taken two hours after dinner or at bedtime. The drugs take four to six weeks to be effective. Avoid drinking grapefruit juice if you're taking statins, as it can interfere with your body's ability to clear some of these drugs from the liver.

Commonly prescribed statins: atorvastatin (*Lipitor*), fluvastatin (*Lescol*), lovastatin (*Mevacor*), pravastatin (*Pravachol*), and simvastatin (*Zocor*).

Fibrates

These drugs are mainly triglyceride-lowering medications. Fibrates reduce the production of triglycerides and remove them from circulation. They do this by stimulating the *lipoprotein lipase*, an enzyme that breaks down lipids in lipoproteins. Studies have shown that fibrates can reduce triglycerides by 20 to 50 percent and increase "good" HDL cholesterol by 10 to 15 percent. Fibrates also mildly reduce LDL cholesterol levels, but the drugs haven't been approved for this purpose.

Most people have few side effects with fibrates, although some experience gastrointestinal problems such as gas or bloating. The drugs also increase the likelihood of developing cholesterol gallstones. They can also magnify the effect of blood-thinning medications.

Commonly prescribed fibrates: Gemfibrozil *(Lopid)* and fenofibrate *(Tricor)*.

Resins

Used for cholesterol lowering for at least 20 years, resins (also called bile acid sequestrants) cause the intestines to absorb less cholesterol from the digestive tract. Bile acids are normally made by the body from cholesterol and pass from the liver into the intestines. Some, however, return to the bloodstream through the intestine wall. Bile acid-binding drugs like resins don't allow the bile acids to return to the bloodstream. They also force more of the cholesterol in the liver to be used to make bile acids, causing less to reach the bloodstream. Over time, this process reduces blood cholesterol. Studies have shown that resins lower LDL cholesterol by 10 to 20 percent. For people with CHD, these drugs are sometimes combined with statins to increase their effectiveness. This combination can often reduce LDL cholesterol by as much as 40 percent.

Resins are available in tablet and powder forms. The powders must be mixed with water or fruit juice and usually taken one to two times a day with meals. Drinking large amounts of water and other liquids can help prevent gastrointestinal problems such as gas, nausea, bloating, and constipation.

Commonly prescribed resins: cholestyramine (*Questran*), colestipol (*Colestid*), and colesevelam (*WelChol*).

Nicotinic Acid

This is the water-soluble B vitamin niacin. Large doses of nicotinic acid can lower triglycerides, lower "bad" LDL cholesterol, and increase "good" HDL cholesterol. It can also change the LDL particles to a larger, less dangerous size. (Nicotinic acid shouldn't be confused with *nicotinamide*, another form of niacin, which doesn't lower cholesterol.)

Nicotinic acid comes in three types: immediate release (*Niacor*), timed release, and extended release (*Niaspan*). In the past, most heart experts recommended the immediate-release type. Now, the longer-acting Niaspan is more often prescribed. Even though it's more expensive, Niaspan has the convenience of once-a-day dosing and fewer side effects. Talk with your doctor about which drug is best for you. Nicotinic acid is widely available without a prescription. However, it should not be used for cholesterol lowering without a doctor's supervision due to potential side effects. Some of the side effects of nicotinic acid include flushing, itching, and stomach upset. Flushing can be lessened by taking an aspirin one hour before.

Taking nicotinic acid with high blood pressure medicines can increase the effects of the blood pressure medication. If you're using this drug combination, it's important that your blood pressure be carefully monitored. Nicotinic acid can also cause liver problems, gout, and an increase in blood sugar levels. If you have diabetes, gout, or stomach ulcers, your doctor may choose a different cholesterol-lowering medication.

Commonly prescribed nicotinic acid: *Niacor, Niaspan.*

Combination Statin and Niacin: *Advicor* (lovastatin and extended release niacin)

Medications to Lower Blood Pressure

ACEs and ARBs

Angiotensin converting enzyme (ACE) inhibitors are a class of drugs that block the formation of angiotensin, a potent chemical that causes tiny arteries to constrict. They are effective in lowering high blood pressure. They help heal the heart muscle after a heart attack and lower the death rate of people with weakened hearts. For people with diabetes, they protect kidney function. ACEs, like other medications, have side effects. The most serious one is kidney failure in people who have narrowing of both kidney arteries, a condition detectable by ultrasound. The most common side effect of ACEs is a dry, hacking cough, which is reversible. ACEs can also cause some people to develop high levels of potassium in the blood. If you take ACEs, your doctor will want to monitor your potassium blood levels and kidney function intermittently.

Commonly prescribed ACEs: benazepril (*Lotensin*), captopril (*Capoten*), fosinopril (*Monopril*), enalapril (*Vasotec*), lisinopril (*Prinivil, Zestril*), ramipril (*Altace*), quinapril (*Accupril*), and trandolapril (*Mavik*).

Angiotensin receptor blockers (ARBs) directly block the effects of angiotensin. They are effective in lowering blood pressure and, for diabetics, for protecting kidney function. ARBs are an alternative medication for people with heart attack or heart failure who cannot use ACEs. The dry cough isn't as big a problem with ARBs.

Commonly prescribed ARBs: candesartan (*Atacand*), irbesartan (*Avapro*), losartan (*Cozaar, Hyzaar*), telmisartan (*Micardis*), and valsartan (*Diovan*).

Diuretics

Commonly called "water pills," these drugs flush excess water and sodium (salt) from the body by increasing urination. This reduces the amount of fluid and sodium in the blood, lowering blood pressure. Diuretics include hydrochlorothiazide (*HCTZ, Hydodiuril*), chlorthalidone (*Hygroton*), indapamide (*Lozol*), furosemide (*Lasix*) and others.

Beta-Blockers

These drugs reduce blood pressure by decreasing heart rate, reducing the strength of the heart's contractions, and relaxing blood vessel walls. For people who have CHD and high blood pressure, a combination of beta-blockers and ACE inhibitors is the preferred treatment. See Anti-anginal medications for more on beta-blockers.

Calcium Channel Blockers

These drugs relax the blood vessels and reduce blood pressure by preventing calcium from entering the muscle cells of the heart. See Anti-anginal medications for more on calcium channel blockers.

Alpha-Blockers

These drugs lower blood pressure by blocking the stimulation of specialized nerves. Alpha-blockers are often used to treat urinary frequency caused by an enlarged prostate gland.

Commonly prescribed alpha-blockers: doxazosin mesylate (*Cardura*), prazosin hydrochloride (*Minipress*), and terazosin hydrochloride (*Hytrin*).

Nerve Inhibitors

The sympathetic nerves extend from the brain to all parts of the body, including the arteries and their tiny branches. Nerve-inhibiting drugs reduce blood pressure by affecting control centers in the brain that keep these nerves from narrowing (constricting) blood vessels. They can be very effective, but their use is limited because they cause fatigue and dry mouth.

Commonly prescribed nerve inhibitors: clonidine (*Catapres*).

Vasodilators

These medications reduce blood pressure by causing the muscle in the walls of the blood vessels, especially the tiny arterioles, to widen or relax. They may also cause the body to retain salt and water and speed heart rate. As a result, they're often prescribed in combination with diuretics and beta-blockers.

Commonly prescribed vasodilators: hydralazine hydro-chloride (*Apresoline*) and minoxidil (*Loniten*).

Getting the Most from Your Medications

Regardless of the type of medication your doctor prescribes, follow these tips to make taking your medications easier, safer, and more effective.

- Let your doctor know about all prescription and over-the-counter (OTC) medications, vitamins, minerals, herbs, and other supplements you're taking.
- Use one pharmacy for all your medications, preferably one that uses computerized drug tracking, to avoid possible dangerous drug interactions.
- Understand how and why you're taking different medications. If you're uncertain, talk with your doctor and/or pharmacist.
- Read labels and any written information that comes with the medicine before taking it. Be sure you read the warnings.
- Ask your doctor or pharmacist before crushing, splitting, or chewing any medication. Some types of medication should only be taken whole.
- If you have side effects or develop new symptoms, talk with your doctor right away. Sometimes the doctor can adjust your medication or have you take it at a different time or in a different way to minimize side effects.
- Take only as much medication as prescribed.
- Don't skip doses or stop taking your medication without your doctor's permission, even if you're feeling better. Some medications need to be tapered off slowly to avoid problems.
- Always talk with your doctor and/or pharmacist before taking over-the-counter medications, vitamins and minerals, or herbal supplements. Some medications

can dangerously interact or become less effective when used with other substances.

- Keep all appointments for tests that monitor your medications. Some drugs have potentially harmful effects and need to be carefully monitored.

- Toss out any medication that has passed its expiration date. Some outdated medications lose their potency; others may become dangerous as they break down over time.

- Never share your medications or take anyone else's medications.

- Organize your medications so that they're easy to take, especially if you take a number of drugs or take them at different times. Pharmacies carry medication reminder devices such as containers that beep, special caps that count how often a prescription bottle has been opened, and computerized drug organizer-dispensers. Putting your medications where you'll see them, keeping them in sectioned containers, taking them at specific times of the day (e.g., meal times), and even checking off a calendar as you take them can help keep you on track.

- Store your medicines in a cool, dry place (unless otherwise directed) in their original containers. Because bathrooms tend to be hot and moist, they are not good storage places for drugs. Keep all medicines away from children.

8

Coronary Angioplasty
and Bypass Surgery

Many people are able to control their coronary heart disease with healthy lifestyle changes and medications. However, if the blockages in your coronary arteries are severe or if you continue to have frequent or disabling chest discomfort (angina) despite medication, you may need to improve the blood supply to your heart. This can be done with coronary angioplasty or with coronary bypass surgery. While anti-anginal medications can decrease the heart's *need* for oxygen and nutrients, angioplasty and bypass surgery can increase the *supply*. Having more blood get to your heart should help reduce or eliminate your angina, reduce your fatigue, and possibly decrease your need for medication. These techniques can improve the quality and even the length of your life.

Coronary Angioplasty

Coronary angioplasty, also called *balloon angioplasty* or *percutaneous transluminal coronary angioplasty (PTCA)*, is a procedure designed to treat the inside surfaces of coronary arteries without having to surgically open the chest. It's designed to widen narrowed coronary arteries using a fine tube that's threaded through an artery to a narrowed blood vessel. Once at the narrowing or blockage, a tiny balloon at the tip of the tube is inflated. As the balloon inflates, it pushes against the plaque, compressing it and enlarging the inside of the artery so that more blood can flow through. Once the inner channel of the artery is enlarged, the balloon is deflated and the catheter is removed.

First performed in 1977, angioplasty has radically changed the treatment for CHD. Before angioplasty, patients were treated either with medications or bypass surgery. The introduction of angioplasty offered a radical new option. However, even though the success rate for these early balloon angioplasties was greater than 90 percent, there were problems. Two to five percent of people who received balloon angioplasty ended up needing emergency bypass surgery when the artery being treated abruptly closed down and threatened a major heart attack. In addition, at least 40 percent of the arteries treated with these early procedures renarrowed (called *restenosis*) within 2 to 6 months.

Today, angioplasty and the tools used to perform it are much more sophisticated. The *interventional cardiologist,* a doctor who specializes in performing angioplasty and other catheter-based surgical interventions, now has tools adapted to treat specific types of narrowings or lesions (much like a carpenter who has a screwdriver for a screw and a hammer for a nail). For instance, to treat calcified plaque the cardiologist uses a diamond-coated burr that spins at 180,000 revolutions per minute in a technique called *rotational atherectomy.* The burr breaks through the plaque and creates a smooth arterial channel. Once the plaque is shattered into tiny bits, the body clears the plaque debris through its own disposal system in the liver, spleen, and bone marrow. In experienced hands, rotational atherectomy has made angioplasty safer for treating complex lesions. Nevertheless, renarrowing rates remained unchanged.

In the early 1990s, *lasers* became popular for "zapping the plaque" during angioplasty. While this technique was first met with great enthusiasm, cardiologists found that it was expensive, offered no better results than other techniques, and was associated with higher complication rates. Laser angioplasty has fallen out of favor and today few cardiologists use it.

In the early to mid-1990s, *directional atherectomy (DCA)*, in which the cardiologist shaves the atherosclerotic plaque and removes it, was widely used. DCA did lower the rates of renarrowing compared with balloon angioplasty, but success rates were very dependent on the technical skills of the cardiologist. Today, DCA has largely been replaced by the use of stents, wire mesh sleeves used to keep narrowed arteries open.

Stents: Propping Arteries Open

The introduction of *stents* was a major breakthrough in angioplasty. Named for Charles R. Stent, the British dentist who developed the concept (he used them to make dental impressions), stents are fine wire-mesh tubes that "prop open" the arteries. They are inserted into the artery with a specially designed catheter. Using stenting, fewer than 1 percent of patients who have angioplasty need emergency bypass surgery during the procedure. In fact, stents have become so popular that they're now used in up to 90 percent of angioplasty procedures.

George is a 37-year-old nonsmoker with a family history of heart disease. He has a mild elevation of his cholesterol, but he feels fine. Worried about his family history of heart disease, George requested an EBT (electron beam tomography), a diagnostic test that measures calcium in the plaque deposits in blood vessels (see chapter 6). The higher the calcium score, the greater the risk for CHD. George's EBT was strongly positive for CHD. His cardiologist performed a nuclear stress test and found George had abnormalities in two areas of his coronary arteries. Cardiac catheterization revealed critical narrowings in two vessels. He was treated with stenting of both vessels. He is now receiving long-term treatment with a statin medication and aspirin.

Renarrowing After Stents

Unfortunately, stents have not been perfect. Scar tissue develops in an average of 20 percent of patients. Because scar tissue grows inward, it can narrow the arteries much like plaque. Although renarrowing can also occur at the treatment site during the first 6 to 12 months from new plaque forming, it is uncommon. Scar-related renarrowing usually occurs within 3 months of the angioplasty, but may happen as late as 1 year later. Restenosis may

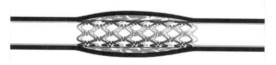

Stents, used to keep arteries open, are made of fine mesh wire. More than one million times a year, physicians treat blockages in arteries and insert stents.

Photo courtesy of Cordis Corporation, a Johnson & Johnson Company.

occur even if you follow all the recommended lifestyle changes and carefully adhere to the prescribed medications. After stenting, some people develop little scars that aren't a problem. Others develop big scars that interfere with blood flow. People at higher risk for renarrowing include: diabetics, those who've had smaller arteries treated, those with longer narrowings, younger patients (30 to 50 years old), and people receiving multiple stents (renarrowing may be related to the amount of metal inserted or to the extent of underlying disease).

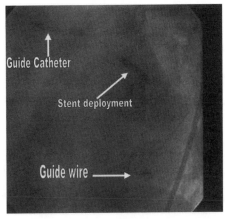

To insert a stent, the stent is attached to a thin catheter that is inserted in a small incision in the groin and guided upwards into the blocked artery.

When stents do renarrow, it is called *instent restenosis.* Treating instent restenosis has had limited success due to a high rate of repeat renarrowing. When conventional balloon angioplasty, rotational atherectomy, or repeat stenting is performed to reopen already treated arteries, 40 to 50 percent of the arteries will renarrow. Rates are somewhat lower if the renarrowing is in a short, focal area, and are higher if the renarrowing involves a longer segment. If a renarrowed artery is treated a second time, it has a 70 percent chance of a repeated renarrowing.

Keeping Stents Open

Intracoronary radiation or *brachytherapy* is now used to treat instent restenosis. The aim of this therapy is to decrease scar tissue formation. Radiation therapy reduces scar formation and restenosis by turning off the natural tendency of the cells to divide and form scar tissue. Two types of radiation are available: *beta* and *gamma*. Both types reduce renarrowing to 20 percent (versus 40 to 50 percent with conventional techniques). In addition to aspirin, people undergoing intracoronary radiation require the anti-clotting drug clopidogrel (Plavix) for at least 1 year.

Drug-coated (Medicated) Stents

An even newer process shows promise. In a landmark clinical trial, stents, coated with medications, reduced the buildup of scar tissue. In one 6-month follow-up study of 238 patients, 26 percent of those with conventional stents showed renarrowing, compared to zero percent of those who received stents that had been coated with medication. By reducing the risk of renarrowing with these and other techniques that are being developed, not only will fewer patients require a return visit to the cath lab, fewer patients may ultimately need bypass surgery.

Other Improvements to Angioplasty

Other technologies have improved the outcomes and safety of angioplasty and stenting. *Intravascular ultrasound (IVUS)* actually gives the doctor images of the inside of your arteries using sound waves. A tiny microphone-like device (transducer) is mounted on the tip of a catheter and inserted into one of the coronary arteries. The ultrasound waves bounce back images of the artery walls and plaque inside the arteries. The images show the degree of calcification, the true size of the artery (more accurate than the angiogram), and how well the stents have been placed.

The *pressure wire*, which is inserted via a catheter, is a diagnostic tool used in the cath lab that can help determine whether a narrowing is severe enough to be treated with angioplasty. It has a sensor that measures the pressure in the artery on both sides of the narrowing. The differences in the pressures can reveal the significance of the blockage.

Different types of protection devices such as balloons with *suction devices, mini-umbrellas,* and *filters on wires* have been designed to help in the treatment of old diseased bypasses. They minimize debris from plaque going downstream and blocking the small arteries of the heart, which can cause heart attacks.

The *AngioJet* is a catheter specialized at breaking up blood clots. Essentially a high-pressure spray, the *AngioJet* can be used during angioplasty with people who have lots of blood clots.

Undergoing an Angioplasty-Stenting Procedure

Angioplasty and stenting are done under local anesthesia and conscious sedation with a relaxant medication similar to Valium. During the procedure, you may feel some angina discomfort—chest heaviness, arm discomfort, shortness of breath—but most people report the procedure isn't painful. The procedure takes ½ hour to 2 hours to complete, depending on the extent of your blockages. In most cases, it requires only an overnight hospital stay.

Before the Procedure

Prior to the procedure, you'll have a chest X-ray, an electrocardiogram performed, and blood tests. You shouldn't eat or drink anything after midnight the night before the procedure. Your doctor will give you medications to decrease blood clotting—aspirin and clopidogrel (Plavix)—and other medications to relax the muscles in your coronary arteries.

The Angioplasty Procedure

During the procedure, your heart rate and rhythm will be monitored. After numbing the area with a local anesthetic, your cardiologist will make a small incision in your groin (less often your arm). Then he or she will insert a long, narrow, hollow tube (catheter) through the artery. Guided by X-ray images the doctor views on a television monitor, the catheter will be moved through the artery to the blocked artery in your heart. This process should be painless. (See chapter 6 for more information on catheterization.)

At this point, the doctor will inject a small amount of contrast dye. This will enable the cardiologist to see the exact location of the blockage. Once the guiding catheter is in the right place, a second, smaller catheter equipped with a deflated balloon (or a burr when appropriate) and a very thin wire (14/1000 of an inch) is inserted into the guide catheter. It, too, is moved through the artery to the blockage. After the wire is threaded across the narrowing, the deflated balloon moves into the blockage area. The doctor inflates the balloon for 30 to 120 seconds to widen the artery and then it is deflated. The doctor may repeat the inflation-deflation several times. During this part of the procedure, you'll likely feel chest pain or pressure. That's because while the balloon is inflated, blood flow through the artery is temporarily blocked. Let the doctor know if you feel pain. In most cases, the pain goes away once the balloon is deflated.

Next, the cardiologist will usually insert a stent(s), the fine wire-mesh tubes for propping open the artery. The stents are mounted on a balloon angioplasty catheter in a collapsed state. It's moved to the blockage area where the balloon is inflated and the stent deployed. The balloon is then deflated and removed, leaving the expanded stent in place. Stents are designed to stay in the artery permanently.

Once the balloon catheter is removed, pictures (angiograms) are taken to see how well blood is flowing through the affected artery. In some cases, results are confirmed with an intravascular ultrasound, an "echo" picture from inside the arteries. If blood is flowing well, the guide catheter will be removed and the sheath (a four-to-six-inch tube) will be sewn into the skin. Once the blood thinners you've been given have been neutralized by the body (about 4 hours), the doctor removes the sheath (leaving the stent in place).

After the Procedure

The medical team will watch your recovery carefully for 12 to 24 hours. Be sure to let the nurses or doctor know if you feel any pain or discomfort following your angioplasty.

Your doctor will order oral, and when indicated, intravenous blood-thinning medication to prevent clot formation. You may also be given nitroglycerine to relax the coronary arteries and calcium antagonists to protect the arteries from spasm.

You'll need to return to your doctor within six months to evaluate how well the procedure is keeping the artery open. The follow-up, which involves a checkup, ECG, and/or nuclear stress tests, can be done in your doctor's office. It's non-invasive and painless. If a stress test indicates it's safe, your doctor may recommend a *cardiac rehabilitation program*—a structured plan of education, exercise, and other lifestyle changes to reduce your cardiac risk factors.

Mike is a 62-year-old who underwent a four-vessel bypass 12 years ago. He went to a cardiologist, saying that on a recent vacation he'd experienced chest discomfort. Mike had reduced his risk factors by quitting smoking, increasing his "good" HDL cholesterol, and getting his blood pressure under control. The physician performed a nuclear stress test and it showed that the bottom of Mike's heart wasn't getting enough blood flow. A diagnostic angiography revealed that three out of four of Mike's original bypasses were still open. One, however, was blocked. The cardiologist treated the blocked artery with three stents, re-establishing a large internal channel. Mike's chest pain was totally eliminated.

How Safe Is Angioplasty?

More than 500,000 angioplasty procedures are performed in the United States every year. Worldwide, it's estimated that more than 1 million are performed annually. For many people, the procedure relieves angina better than medication alone. With the availability and use of stents, success rates for treating arteries that are less than 100 percent blocked exceed 95 percent. The success of treating total blockages with angioplasty depends largely on how long the artery has been 100 percent blocked. If the artery has been completely blocked for less than three months, the angioplasty success rate is 80 percent. It drops to less than 50 percent if the artery has been completely blocked for more than three months.

Angioplasty is easier and less invasive than coronary artery bypass graft surgery (CABG). It doesn't involve general anesthesia, it's less expensive, hospital stays are shorter, and recovery time is faster. Major complications are unusual. In addition, if the procedure needs to be repeated, the risks are no higher than the initial procedure. (A repeat bypass operation is riskier than the first)

Potential Risks

Angioplasty is relatively safe. The risk of death from angioplasty is less than 1 percent. The risk of having a minor heart attack during the procedure is 2 to 6 percent, a major heart attack less than 1 percent. The need for emergency bypass surgery is less than 1 percent. The incidence of heart attack, stroke, and the death rate following angioplasty is higher for women than for men. This may be because women who undergo the procedure tend to be older and have a higher incidence of high blood pressure, diabetes, high blood choles-terol, and other health problems than men who undergo the procedure.

In addition to the rare risks of heart attack, death, and stroke, other complications may occur. These complications are usually treatable. They include:

- All possible complications related to cardiac catheterization
- Injury or puncture of the artery during insertion of the catheter
- Increased risk of clot formation inside the artery
- Blockages made worse (e.g., a 90 percent renarrowing after treatment of a 50 percent blockage)

Your physician must advise you of the risk of not treating your CHD blockages weighed against the risk of complications.

Who Is a Candidate for Angioplasty?

Previously, angioplasty was performed only on people who had one severely blocked artery. Now, due to advances in the procedure, doctors are using angioplasty on people with severe and even multiple blockages. Studies show that the procedure provides more complete relief than medication alone for people with angina. Depending on where the blockages are located, angioplasty is equivalent to bypass surgery in providing relief from angina, in risk of heart attack, and in long-term survival rates. The exceptions are diabetics who have significant blockages in the main artery to the front of the heart (left descending artery or LAD). At least for now, these individuals are better suited for bypass surgery.

Whether angioplasty or the more invasive coronary bypass surgery is right for you is a decision you and your doctor will have to make together, depending on:

- Where your blockages are
- How many blockages you have
- How extensive the blockages are

- Your age
- Your overall health
- How well your heart is functioning
- How hardened (calcified) your plaques are

You may *not* be a candidate for angioplasty if:

- The plaque is located in an area inaccessible by catheter (too far or in a curve in the artery)
- The plaque is severely calcified (In skilled hands, rotational atherectomy is usually successful.)
- Plaque is in the left main coronary artery
- Blockage is complete in one or more coronary arteries (especially if the artery has been blocked for a long time)

If you're not a candidate for angioplasty, coronary bypass surgery may be more appropriate for you.

Coronary Artery Bypass Graft Surgery (CABG)

Coronary bypass, also known as *coronary artery bypass graft surgery* (*CABG*, pronounced "cabbage"), may be an option for blockages that can't be adequately treated with angioplasty. This might include people who have arteries that are chronically totally blocked, narrowing in all the coronary arteries, and/or narrowing in the left main coronary artery. Also, people who are diabetic and have narrowings in the artery that supplies the front of the heart (left anterior descending artery or LAD) have better results with bypass surgery, especially if the narrowings involve long segments.

Both angioplasty and bypass surgery increase blood supply to the heart. Angioplasty fixes the artery in its natural channel by removing the blockage from the artery. In contrast, bypass surgery goes *around* the problem arteries, much like a construction detour. The bypass procedure involves taking a piece of blood vessel, usually from the chest and/or leg, and stitching it onto the blocked artery beyond the narrowing. In many cases, more than one artery is blocked, requiring multiple bypasses. The procedure takes 2 to 5 hours, depending on the number of bypasses and the complexity of the surgery.

Who Is a Candidate for Bypass Surgery?

In general, bypass surgery is used when coronary blockages are severe and widespread, especially if three arteries are blocked or the blockages occur at critical locations in the heart's circulatory system. Because bypass is a major operation, your doctor will recommend it only after careful consideration. In addition to assessing the location and extent of your blockages, your doctor will consider the overall health of your heart, your age, and other non-heart health problems you may have.

You may have a choice of undergoing angioplasty or bypass surgery. Ask your doctor about the risks and benefits of each. You may also want to get a second or even a third opinion before making your decision. You *may* be a candidate for bypass surgery if:

- Your angina is debilitating and interferes with normal functions of daily life

- Two or all three main coronary arteries are narrowed 75 percent or more (Some people with CHD in only one vessel may also benefit.)
- The left main coronary artery is 70 percent or more narrowed (50 percent in some cases)
- You have poor function of the left ventricle, the heart's main pumping station, which may improve with a renewed blood supply
- You have a very abnormal exercise or nuclear test despite no symptoms
- You're not a good candidate for angioplasty/stenting
- You've already undergone a catheter treatment that's been unsuccessful
- Bypasses from a previous operation have closed

Before Surgery

Once you're admitted to the hospital, you'll be given blood and urine tests, a chest X-ray, ECG, and other tests. Unless you've already had angiograms taken, a diagnostic cardiac catheterization or angiography will be performed. The images will serve as a road map that enables your surgeon to know where to place the bypasses. The night before your surgery, you'll also take a shower with a special soap to decrease the risk of infection.

You'll probably take your regular medications, but you should ask your doctor first. Your doctor will likely have you not take aspirin or other blood-thinning medications to avoid the risk of bleeding during and immediately following the surgery. (Urgent bypass surgeries are frequently done while the patient is taking these medications and often require blood transfusions.) A nurse will prepare you for surgery by shaving your chest and legs. About an hour before surgery, you'll be given a sedative to help you relax. Once you're in the operating room, the anesthesiologist will give you a general anesthetic to put you to sleep. He or she will insert a special intravenous line to help monitor your blood pressure and the pressure inside your lungs during the operation.

The Bypass Procedure

Your surgeon will expose your heart by making an incision through the middle of the chest and through the breastbone. Once the heart is exposed, you'll be put on the *heart-lung bypass*, or *pump oxygenator*. Specialized health professionals called *perfusionists* operate this machine. The heart-lung machine takes venous blood that's returning from the body and oxygenates it like the lungs would. Then it pumps the blood into the aorta downstream from the heart, where it flows to all the organs. While you're on the heart-lung bypass, your heart is stopped and blood doesn't flow to it (what surgeons call a "bloodless field"). This allows the surgeon to work precisely on the heart while it's not moving. To ensure the heart isn't damaged during this time, the heart is cooled and chemicals are added to reduce its need for oxygen. (During off-pump surgery, which doesn't use the heart-lung machine, blood flows through the coronary arteries to the heart throughout the operation.)

While the heart is stopped, the bypass arteries and/or veins are delicately sewn into place. The average is three or four bypasses. Once the grafts are in place, the heart is rewarmed. The surgeon uses electric shock to restart the heart and then closes the incisions.

Harvesting Blood Vessels for Bypass

Many people are concerned about the blood vessels used in bypass. Won't you miss them? Won't the area from which they're taken suffer? No. The arteries or veins used in bypass aren't essential. Removing, or "harvesting" them doesn't significantly impact the blood flow from where they're taken. The internal mammary artery (thoracic artery), located on the inside chest wall, is used in 90 percent of bypass procedures. We have two mammary arteries: one on the left and one on the right side of the chest. (The right mammary artery is used less in bypass). The mammary arteries tend to stay open longer than other blood vessels that can be used. When a mammary artery is used, an additional incision is not required, and the surgeon usually doesn't have to entirely remove it. Instead, he or she reconnects the downstream part of the mammary artery to the coronary artery, bypassing the blockage.

Most bypasses use some of the superficial vein that runs down the inside of the leg (saphenous vein). Sometimes veins are taken from both legs. A specially trained physician assistant or an assisting surgeon will make another incision on the inside of one or both legs to remove the vein. Once the vein

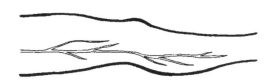

When additional veins are needed for by-pass surgery, they are often taken from the saphenous vein that runs down the side of the leg.

is removed, one end of it is connected to the aorta and the other to the coronary artery downstream from the blockage. Less commonly, veins may be taken from the backs of the legs or arms. Sometimes the artery that supplies blood to the hand (radial artery) is used if the other hand artery (ulnar artery) can provide an adequate supply of blood to the hand. If needed, an artery in the abdomen can be redirected and used as a bypass graft.

Recovery from Bypass Surgery

After surgery, you'll be taken to a cardiac surgery recovery area or intensive care unit for 24 to 36 hours. Small tubes in your chest and arms will remain in place for 24 hours. They allow the doctors to check for internal bleeding, give drugs and fluids, withdraw blood samples, drain off fluid, and continuously monitor your blood pressure. Small patches (electrodes) on your chest let the staff monitor your heart's rate and rhythm with the ECG. A breathing tube (*endotracheal tube*) that goes through the mouth into your windpipe will help you breathe. It's usually removed within the first 24 hours.

After the first 24 hours following surgery, recovery is usually fairly quick. You should be alert and able to eat and walk. If you've had one or more veins removed from your legs, you may need to wear elastic support stockings to help circulation and reduce swelling. About 20 percent of people who've undergone bypass surgery require a blood transfusion following surgery. Thirty to forty percent develop erratic heart rhythm problems (atrial fibrillation) that require special care. A few develop infection at the wound site. Barring these complications, you should be able to leave the hospital in five or six days.

You'll need to return in a week or so to have any external stitches or staples removed from your chest. If you have leg stitches, they'll need to stay in a few days longer. Most people

Common Sites for Bypass Grafts

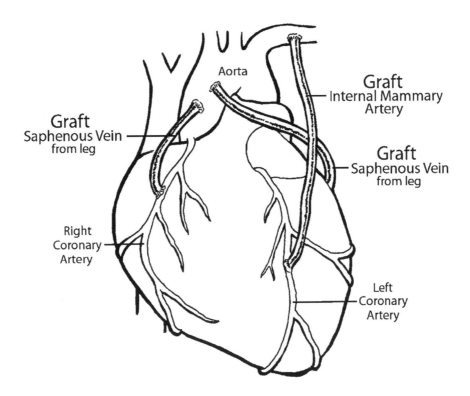

Bypass grafting is performed under magnification with hair-fine sutures. One end of each graft is sewn to the aorta; the other end is sewn to the artery below the blockage.

tions, you should be able to leave the hospital in five or six days.

Your surgical wounds should heal within six weeks or so. If you have a sedentary job, you'll likely be able to return to work in about four weeks. If you have a physically demanding occupation, you may need to wait six weeks or longer. Your doctor will usually recommend a monitored exercise program. You may participate in the program while you are working in a light job. However, if you have a job requiring heavy physical labor, you'll probably need to complete the monitored exercise program before returning to work.

During recovery, it's important to avoid heavy lifting and take time to build up your endurance. You can't drive for six weeks. At first you'll likely feel weak and tired. That's understandable, considering that a week in bed shrinks muscle strength by 15 percent. It also takes a lot of energy for your body to heal itself. Walking is a great way to regain your strength and energy. You'll want to keep an eye out for warning signs of infection, fluid retention, or problems with your bypasses, including:

- Redness or drainage at the incision site
- Fever
- Chills
- Increasing fatigue
- Weight gain over five pounds in a few days
- Changes in heart rate or rhythms (palpitations or skipped beats)
- Swollen ankles (Often the leg from which the vein was taken swells more, making the legs feel unequal.)

Six years ago, Lou, a 49-year-old executive, had a small heart attack and underwent an urgent five-vessel bypass surgery. After the surgery, he stopped smoking and started exercising. Recently, he'd returned to his old ways. He started smoking again, stopped exercising, and he'd gained weight. He noticed he was short of breath, especially when he walked in cold weather. A nuclear stress test showed Lou had developed a new small abnormality. He underwent an EBA, a non-invasive electron beam angiogram. It revealed the two mammary arterial grafts and two of his three venous bypasses were open. However, the third venous graft contained the small narrowing seen on the nuclear test. Lou's cardiologist recommended that he be treated with medication and lifestyle changes. Realizing that CHD is a lifelong problem, Lou once again altered his lifestyle.

Is Coronary Bypass Surgery Safe?

Coronary artery bypass is major surgery. It carries risks. The biggest risk, of course, is dying. The overall risk of dying from bypass surgery is 1 to 2 percent. For women, it's slightly higher. It still means that 95 to 99 percent of people who undergo bypass surgery will survive. If you must undergo the surgery during an emergency situation such as a heart attack, your risk of dying increases to 5 to 8 percent. Fortunately, emergency surgery is less common than it was prior to the availability of stents. The risks are also higher for people who are older or who have extensive scarring from previous heart attacks.

Coronary artery bypass substantially improves symptoms in 90 percent of those who undergo the operation. Sometimes renarrowings develop in the bypasses themselves. Ten years after surgery, one-third of venous bypasses are closed, one-third are narrowed, and one-third remain widely open. The results with mammary artery bypasses are better—a full 96 percent remain open after 10 years. On average, the 5-year survival rate for men who have undergone bypass is 90 to 94 percent. For women, the 5-year survival rate is 87 to 91 percent. This survival rate means that an individual will be alive *at least* five years later.

Newer Bypass Techniques

Coronary bypass surgery has traditionally required the use of a heart-lung machine (*pump oxygenator*). During surgery, the heart-lung machine keeps your blood flowing and oxygenated, while allowing the surgeon to stop your heart so that the bypasses can be precisely connected.

Recently, less invasive forms of bypass have become available. One, called *minimally invasive direct coronary artery bypass* or *MIDCAB,* has become popular because it has been shown that bypass can be done without the heart-lung machine and it requires a shorter hospital stay than the standard surgery. In MIDCAB, a smaller incision is made in the chest directly over the artery or arteries to be bypassed. An advantage to MIDCAB is that it avoids the use of the heart-lung machine because it's performed on a beating heart. The surgeon detaches an artery, usually from inside the chest, and reattaches it to the clogged artery. MIDCAB is generally designed for use when only one or two arteries need to be bypassed. *OPCAB* or *off-pump coronary artery bypass*, is used more often than MIDCAB. The chest incision is the same as in a standard bypass operation, but the heart-lung machine isn't used. The cardiac surgeon works on the heart while it's beating, often attaching several bypasses. Both off-pump procedures require that the operating room be ready to go on full heart-lung bypass if complications occur.

At a few centers, surgeons are attempting another limited-access surgery, *port-access coronary artery bypass* or *PACAB*. In PACAB, the surgeon makes small holes in the chest. Instruments are passed through the ports to perform the bypass as the surgeon watches the surgery on video monitors. Arteries from the chest or veins from the legs (saphenous veins) are used to bypass clogged heart vessels. This technique does require the heart to be stopped and blood to be pumped through the heart-lung machine.

These newer procedures are being carefully evaluated. A recent major comparison of people eligible for both techniques—heart-lung machine and off-pump—showed the success of the bypasses were similar. However, techniques that didn't use the heart-lung machine had fewer complications. Off-pump surgeries had lower rates of stroke, short-term memory loss, bleeding, shorter hospital stays, and required fewer transfusions.

Off-pump bypass now accounts for 20 percent of the bypasses performed. It's especially being used in people 75 years and older, a group that's more at risk for stroke. Some doctors are ordering an MRI of the aorta to look for plaque before deciding whether to use on- or off-bypass surgery. The presence of plaque in the aorta may signal a higher risk for stroke, in which case an off-pump technique may be a better choice. Though off-pump techniques are gaining favor, studies are still going on to determine who is best suited for off-pump bypass.

Other Technologies

For people with chronically blocked arteries, angioplasty isn't an option. For those with artery problems downstream from bypasses, coronary bypass surgery can't be used. For these individuals, other technologies need to be considered. Let's look at a few of these approaches.

Transmyocardial Revascularization (TMR)

Transmyocardial revascularization or *TMR* is a technique used to treat chest pain. In TMR, the surgeon makes an incision in the left chest, exposing the heart. Then he or she uses a laser to drill 20 to 40 one-millimeter holes into the heart's pumping chamber. Bleeding from the holes stops within a few minutes. The idea was that oxygenated blood on the inside of the heart would give the heart some nourishment and the procedure might stimulate new blood vessels to grow (a process called *angiogenesis*).

We aren't sure why TMR relieves chest pain. Some believe TMR increases blood supply. However, others think the procedure simply destroys nerves in the area so that the heart is numb to the pain.

Regardless of how TMR works, as many as 80 to 90 percent of people who've undergone the procedure have had at least 50 percent improvement in symptoms for the first year. Other research suggests TMR is effective for longer periods of time. In one study, 60 percent of patients who'd undergone TMR had chest pain relief for at least five years. TMR may be combined with bypass surgery for pain relief for people with widespread blockages. However, so far, studies of TMR have not been well controlled and therefore its effectiveness is questionable.

Percutaneous Transmyocardial Revascularization (PTMR)

Another treatment for chest pain that's a non-surgical form of TMR is *percutaneous transmyocardial revascularization (PTMR)*, or *direct myocardial revascularization (DMR)*. It doesn't require general anesthesia and requires only an overnight stay. The cardiologist passes a laser in a catheter to the heart. The laser, inserted on the tip of the catheter, places holes in the inner thickness of the heart. However, the results haven't been promising. Research shows that groups of patients who thought they'd received this laser treatment (the placebo group) showed the same improvement as those who actually did receive the laser treatment. Based on this research, this treatment can't be recommended.

Hope for the Future

Gene Therapy

One of the newer areas for treating disease, including coronary heart disease, is *gene therapy*. Researchers believe that many diseases may be a result of defects in one or more genes. Most likely, CHD is caused by a combination of environmental and genetic factors. For instance, your high cholesterol may be caused by your heredity along with a combination of unhealthy diet and other lifestyle factors. Gene therapy may be able to deal with the hereditary contribution to your disease.

Gene therapy involves introducing genetic material into cells. For instance, doctors might insert new genes into vascular cells to prevent them from becoming renarrowed. Or, in areas where blood supply isn't adequate, doctors may be able to use genes to grow new blood vessels. These techniques are being tested in the cath lab and in the operating room using proteins, inactivated viruses (which program the body to make new vessels), or stem cells.

One study conducted on people with leg bypass surgeries who received gene therapy found that the gene therapy helped prevent restenosis of the grafted blood vessels. The vein to be grafted was bathed in a fluid containing small bits of DNA, the material from which genes are made. This material causes the genes that can lead to abnormal cell growth and renarrowing to short-circuit. Those who had the gene therapy had 50 percent fewer renarrowing problems than those who had the bypass surgery alone.

In another study, researchers at Cornell University injected genetic material (in this case an inactive virus) that coded for vascular endothelial growth factor (VEGF) directly into the oxygen-starved hearts of patients. Most patients said they had less chest pain following the injection. Additionally, new blood cells grew in response to the therapy, improving blood flow to the heart and heart-wall functioning.

In the future, gene therapy may be used alone as therapy or used in combination with other more conventional treatments such as balloon angioplasty or coronary bypass surgery. Gene therapy offers exciting new hope for treating CHD.

9

Lifestyle Treatments for Coronary Heart Disease

Medical science has made great strides in treating coronary heart disease. New and better medications are more effective and have fewer side effects (see chapter 7). Surgical interventions are more sophisticated than ever, leading to fewer complications and better outcomes. However, heart authorities, including the National Heart, Lung, and Blood Institute, agree that changing unhealthy lifestyle habits is still the single most important thing you can do to stop the disease from progressing. There's evidence that making heart-healthy lifestyle changes such as changing what you eat, your activity level, and how you deal with stress may prevent a heart attack and may even reverse the narrowing of your arteries.

Lower Your High Blood Cholesterol

As you know, having high blood cholesterol is a major risk factor for CHD and heart attack. High levels of "bad" LDL cholesterol and triglycerides and low levels of "good" HDL cholesterol play a major role in the development of CHD and heart attacks. If you have high cholesterol, your doctor will likely recommend changes in your diet and other lifestyle modifications. You may also need to take cholesterol-lowering medication.

You can control several things that affect your blood cholesterol:

- **What you eat.** If you're eating a lot of saturated fat, dietary cholesterol, and too many calories (leading to excess weight), chances are you have high cholesterol.
- **Weight.** Being overweight can make your "bad" LDL cholesterol go up and your "good" HDL cholesterol go down.
- **Physical activity.** Being inactive makes you a candidate for high LDL and low HDL.

What's a Heart-Healthy Diet?

A *heart-healthy diet* is an integral part of getting your high blood cholesterol under control. Research has shown that a heart-healthy diet can not only slow the progression of plaque, it can also stabilize and even reverse atherosclerosis. Research shows that dietary changes can reduce total and LDL cholesterol levels by 10 to 15 percent, which translates to as much as a 20 to 30 percent reduction in heart disease risk.

If you're like most Americans, your diet contains 35 to 45 percent fat and 400 to 500 milligrams per day of cholesterol. That's way too much fat and cholesterol for a healthy heart. In Japan, where they eat a low-fat diet that typically contains 10 to 20 percent fat, CHD and high blood cholesterol are rare.

Here are some general guidelines for a heart-healthy diet.

Eat less total dietary fat. The American Heart Association (AHA) recommends getting no more than 30 percent of your total daily calories from fat. The National Cholesterol Education Program (NCEP) of the National Institutes of Health recommends 25 to 35 percent of your total calories come from fat.

Eat less saturated fat. Saturated fat is the biggest culprit in raising blood cholesterol, especially "bad" LDL cholesterol. Saturated fats come from animal products such as meats, cheeses, butter, and whole dairy products. The AHA recommends no more than 8 to 10 percent of your daily fat calories come from saturated fats. For those with heart disease, both the AHA and NCEP recommend 7 percent or less of your daily fat calories come from saturated fats.

Choose polyunsaturated and monounsaturated fats over saturated fats. When it comes to the heart, not all fats are created equal. Polyunsaturated fats (safflower, sesame, sunflower, corn, and soybean oil, and oils from nuts) and monounsaturated fats (olive, canola, peanut, avocado oils) are made from vegetable sources. Both types may lower blood cholesterol when used in place of saturated fats. Monounsaturated fat, in particular, has been associated with lowering LDL cholesterol.

The AHA recommends up to 10 percent of your fat calories come from polyunsaturated fats and up to 15 percent come from monounsaturated fat. New guidelines from NCEP recommend up to 10 percent polyunsaturated fat calories and up to 20 percent monounsaturated fat calories.

131

Limit dietary cholesterol. Dietary cholesterol is found in foods from animals (meat, fish, poultry, eggs, and dairy products). These foods are also sources of saturated fat. Egg yolks and organ meats like liver are loaded with cholesterol. Foods from plant sources such as fruits, vegetables, grains, cereals, nuts, and seeds contain no cholesterol.

The AHA recommends limiting dietary cholesterol to no more than 300 milligrams per day for men and 220 to 260 milligrams per day for women. For those who've had a coronary event, the AHA recommends less than 200 milligrams per day. The NCEP recommends no more than 200 milligrams per day.

Choose foods high in complex carbohydrates. Foods that are high in carbohydrates (starches and sugars) such as rice, pasta, and potatoes are loaded with vitamins and minerals and are actually lower in calories than high-fat foods. The AHA suggests carbohydrates make up 55 to 60 percent of the calories in your daily diet. The NCEP recommendation of 50-60 percent carbohydrates is similar.

Eat foods rich in fiber. The indigestible parts of plant foods, fiber can help lower cholesterol and help keep you "regular." Some studies indicate eating fiber-rich foods may lower blood cholesterol. Additionally, fiber may be instrumental in preventing colon cancer, hemorrhoids, and in the development of painful, sac-like pouches in the intestine (diverticula). It also makes you feel fuller, which can help prevent overeating. Fiber is found in fresh fruits and vegetables and whole grains. The AHA suggests getting plenty of fiber by eating five to nine servings per day of fruits and vegetables and six or more servings of grain products, including whole grains. The NCEP recommends eating 20 to 30 grams of fiber each day.

Choose lean protein. Limit protein to no more than 6 ounces per day and choose leaner cuts of meat, chicken, and fish or fatty meats. Beans, legumes, and soy products such as tofu are good, low-fat sources of protein. Opt for lower fat dairy products.

Balance calories with output. Don't overeat. Eating more calories than you burn leads to becoming overweight, a major CHD and heart attack risk factor.

Limit alcohol. Drinking a small amount of alcohol is associated with fewer heart-related problems. However, most heart authorities don't recommend taking up drinking alcohol if you don't drink. Alcohol abuse is associated with increases

Heart-Healthy Dietary Guidelines

Nutrient	AHA Recommendation	NCEP Recommendation
Total fat	Up to 30%	25-35%
Saturated fat	8-10%/7% or less **	79% or less
Polyunsaturated fat	Up to 10%	Up to 10%
Monounsaturated fat	Up to 15%	Up to 20%
Cholesterol	<300 mg/<200 mg **	< 200 mg
Carbohydrate	55-60%	50-60%
Fiber	5-9 servings fruits/vegetables, 6+ servings grains	20-30 grams
Protein	No more than 6 oz. per day	15% of total calories
Total calories	Balance with output to avoid becoming overweight	Balance with output to avoid becoming overweight

(** Lower values are for those who have diagnosed CHD or have had a coronary event.)

in a number of health problems, including high blood pressure and an elevation in triglycerides (both are CHD risk factors). If you do enjoy an occasional drink, limit your intake to no more than two alcoholic drinks per day for men, one per day for women.

How Much Fat Can You Have?

If you're following the 30% total fat/10% saturated fat guidelines, here's how much fat you can have based on the total calories you eat daily.

Total Calories	30% Total Fat**	10% Saturated Fat
1,500 calories	450 calories or 50 grams	150 calories or 17 grams
1,800 calories	540 calories or 60 grams	180 calories or 20 grams
2,000 calories	600calories or 67 grams	200 calories or 22 grams
2,500 calories	750 calories or 83 grams	250 calories or 28 grams

** Each gram of fat = 9 calories

Other Diets

The AHA's eating plan and the NCEP's dietary recommendations aren't the only heart-healthy diets you can follow. Let's look at a few of the more popular heart-healthy diets:

Mediterranean-Style Diets

Studies have associated Mediterranean-style diets with a lower risk of heart disease. In general, fewer people from the Mediterranean countries of Spain, Greece, and Italy die from CHD than people in northern Europe or the United States.

Since diets vary among peoples of the Mediterranean countries and even among regions within countries, there's no single diet we can label as *the* Mediterranean diet. Generally speaking, Mediterranean diets are rich in fruits, vegetables, cereals, fish, and beans. Mediterranean diets are also higher in total fat than other heart-healthy diets. However, the fats are primarily monounsaturated (mostly olive oil) and omega-3 fats, those found in cold-water fish such as herring, salmon, tuna, and mackerel and in soybean and canola oils.

The Mediterranean-style diet is heart-healthy because it contains a number of protective nutrients: antioxidants such as vitamin E from fruits and vegetables, monounsaturated fatty acids from olive oil, and polyunsaturated omega-3 fatty acids from fish. Studies have shown that monounsaturated and polyunsaturated fats may make the platelets (clotting elements in the blood) less sticky and therefore less likely to clot. For people who are diabetic, these fats can also help lower blood cholesterol (when substituted for saturated fats) better than the high-carbohydrate diets advocated by the AHA and NCEP.

Asian Diet

Like the Mediterranean-style diet, there is no single Asian diet. However, research shows that people from Asian countries who eat a traditional diet have low rates of chronic disease, including CHD. That's because most Asian cuisine emphasizes plant-based foods, including vegetables, rice, beans, soy foods, nuts, seeds, and tea. The traditional Asian diet is low in fat, includes moderate amounts of fish, poultry, and eggs, and is low in red meats, cheese, and yogurt. In fact, in many Asian countries, traditional cuisine doesn't include dairy products at all.

Ornish Diet

Dean Ornish, M.D., director of the Preventive Medicine Research Institute in Sausalito, California, and author of *Dr. Dean Ornish's Program for Reversing Heart Disease*, published studies in the early 1990s showing that a comprehensive program of very low-fat, vegetarian eating, regular exercise, and stress management can actually *reverse* atherosclerosis in some patients with heart disease. Overall, Dr. Ornish found that the plaque in patients who adhered to less stringent diets (such as those advocated by the AHA and NCEP) continued to increase. Those on the AHA and NCEP diets experienced more than twice as many coronary events as those on the Ornish program.

The Ornish Diet, also called the "Reversal Diet," is a vegetarian diet that restricts total fat to 10 percent. It emphasizes fruits, vegetables, beans, whole grains, and nonfat dairy products and contains no meat, fish, poultry, or added fat.

Dr. Ornish's research has shown that over time even severe atherosclerosis can be reversed without the use of drugs in some patients. While a very low-fat vegetarian diet may not be right for everyone, Ornish's diet offers an alternative for reducing CHD risk.

Lose Excess Weight

Being overweight isn't just a cosmetic problem. It is a risk factor for CHD, diabetes, high blood cholesterol, high triglycerides, and high blood pressure. Experts estimate that 75 percent of all high blood pressure is related to excessive weight. Carrying excess weight puts a strain on your heart, making it work harder, even at rest. It also increases total cholesterol, "bad" LDL cholesterol, and triglycerides and decreases "good"

HDL cholesterol, all contributing to the buildup of atherosclerotic plaque. If you carry your extra weight around your waist, the risk to your heart is even greater. It's no wonder the American Heart Association calls excessive weight a major risk factor for heart disease.

Losing even a small amount— 5 to 10 percent of your body weight—can help decrease your risks. Losing as little as 11 to 22 pounds can decrease your risk of developing high blood pressure by as much as 25 percent. It can also help lower your "bad" LDL cholesterol and triglyc-erides and increase your "good" HDL cholesterol.

Eating only 50 excess calories per day results in 5 pounds of weight gain a year.

The How-to of Losing Weight

Work with your doctor. Have a checkup before you begin a weight-loss program. Your doctor can help you develop a sensible weight-loss program.

Set a reasonable goal. Your initial weight loss goal should be 10 percent of your current weight. Once you achieve this goal, set another goal, if needed.

Allow enough time. Slow and steady is the best path to permanent weight loss. Six months is a reasonable timeline for losing 10 percent of your current weight.

Aim for 1 to 2 pounds per week. Most women can lose 1 to 2 pounds a week by eating 1,200 to 1,500 calories per day. Most men can lose this amount by eating 1,500 to 1,800 calories per day. Talk with your doctor about the right amount of calories per day for you.

Accept responsibility. You are the only one who can make the changes in your diet and exercise regimen to lose weight. Are you ready to accept personal responsibility and reduce your risk for heart disease?

Cut the fat. Gram for gram, fat contains more than twice the calories of protein or carbohydrates (9 calories/gram for fat; 4 calories/gram for protein and carbohydrates). That's why cutting dietary fat cuts calories.

Choose a balanced approach. The low-saturated-fat, low-calorie guidelines in this chapter are also terrific for losing weight. Choose nutrient-rich, low-calorie foods such as raw vegetables, some fruits, and complex carbohydrates (rice, pasta, whole-grain breads and cereals).

Avoid crash or fad diets. They may promise quick results, but they don't promote lifestyle changes that will enable you to maintain weight loss for a lifetime.

Take a multivitamin. Take a daily vitamin and mineral supplement to ensure you're meeting the minimum daily requirements.

Drink plenty of water. Drinking six to eight glasses of water a day is not only good for you, it'll help fill you up.

Keep a diary. Recording everything you eat can help avoid "cheating." Also use your diary to record your weight loss, how you're feeling, and your exercise routine.

Weigh once per week. Weighing yourself every day is discouraging. The changes usually reflect only fluctuations in water retention.

Watch for danger zones. All of us have food triggers—people, places, and things that make us want to overeat or indulge in high-fat, high-calorie foods. Identify and avoid your food triggers.

Slow down. It takes 15 minutes or so after eating for your brain to "register" with fullness signals. Slow down and take your time. Eating lots of high-fiber foods like vegetables can also make you feel fuller.

Reward yourself. As you achieve mini-goals in your weight loss plan, reward yourself with small, non-food rewards (e.g., take yourself to a movie, buy a music CD or book).

Exercise. A program of regular exercise can help you eat less, increase the calories you burn, and help reduce other CHD risk factors. It can also decrease abdominal fat, the most dangerous type. Regular exercise is key to maintaining weight loss. Exercise experts say that for weight loss, how hard you exercise isn't as important as for how long. For instance, the calorie expenditure per unit time of exercise varies according to how rigorous the exercise is. As you lose fat and your body becomes more efficient at using calories, you'll need to increase how much you exercise to lose further body fat. For the most effective weight loss, start by walking 30 minutes (or build up to 30 minutes) three times per week. Over time, build up to 45 minutes a day at least five times a week. Your permanent exercise/weight-management goal should be to exercise at least 30 minutes or more a day most (preferably all) days of the week.

Exercise Regularly

As noted previously, regular exercise is key to reducing high blood cholesterol and losing and keeping off excess weight. Physical inactivity is clearly a risk factor for heart disease. By exercising regularly, you can cut your risk of having a heart attack by nearly 50 percent. Even if you've already had a heart attack, regular physical activity can lower the risk of having a second heart attack. Regular exercise:

- **Lowers blood pressure and helps prevent the development of high blood pressure.** If you have mild high blood pressure and you exercise, your blood pressure will drop to healthier levels for 8 to 12 hours after exercising. In some individuals, regular exercise is as effective as medication for lowering high blood pressure—without negative side effects.

- **Lowers heart rate, allowing the heart to pump more efficiently.** Exercise also helps reduce dangerous swings in heart rate.

- **Improves blood cholesterol.** Exercise can drop your total blood cholesterol by as much as 24 percent and "bad" LDL cholesterol by 10 percent. Exercise can also increase "good" HDL cholesterol by 6 percent. The amount of activity needed for these improvements is moderate (e.g. a 30-minute walk most days of the week).

- **Lowers the body's tendency to produce dangerous blood clots,** a key factor in heart attack and stroke. Regular exercise raises the levels of plasminogen, an anticoagulant that may help prevent blood clots.

- **Burns body fat.** As you know, excess fat is a risk factor for heart disease, high blood pressure, diabetes, and other serious health problems. Exercise helps the body use insulin more efficiently. Exercise helps the body clear excess sugar from the blood and makes it more sensitive to insulin, reducing the risk of diabetes.
- **Reduces stress,** a potential contributor to heart disease risk.

Is It Safe to Exercise?

For most people, even those with heart disease, the health benefits of exercise far outweigh the risks. One study published in *Circulation* found elderly men aged 71 to 93 cut their risk of heart attack by 50 percent simply by walking about two miles a day. Another study found that people who exercised following a heart attack lowered their risk of having a second attack by 60 percent.

However, if you have a chronic health condition or other serious health problem, your doctor may want to outline some special exercise precautions. See your doctor for a pre-exercise checkup if you:

- Have heart or lung disease, arthritis, or kidney disease
- Have CHD risk factors (smoking, high blood pressure, diabetes, etc.)
- Are taking medicine for high blood pressure or a heart condition
- Are 40 or older
- Are overweight
- Have a family history of early CHD

If you have heart disease, your doctor may want you to undergo an exercise stress test to determine how much exercise is safe for you. It can help you know what maximum heart rate during exercise is safe for you (you can monitor heart rate during exercise with a pulsemeter). For those who've had a heart attack or undergone angioplasty or bypass surgery, your doctor should prescribe cardiac rehabilitation, which features carefully supervised physical activity.

The most common risk of physical activity is joint or muscle injury. This usually happens when you start exercising too hard or for too long, especially if you haven't been active for some time. Most of these injuries can be prevented by warming up before and cooling down after exercise and building up stamina slowly.

Heat exhaustion or heatstroke can be another problem if you're exercising during hot, humid weather. Both can be avoided with a little common sense—drink plenty of water, exercise less intensely on hot days, try to exercise during a cooler time of day, and watch for warning signs such as dizziness, headache, and nausea.

Rarely, people have died while exercising. This can be a big fear for someone who has heart disease. For people who have heart disease, following your doctor's orders and gradually building up your condition will reduce the risk of exercise-related problems. If you're considered high risk for heart attack, you should exercise in a monitored facility with staff who are trained in cardiac resuscitation.

The How-to of Exercise Success

Go slowly. Start slowly and build up. If you're inactive, you may want to begin with a 10-to-15-minute walk, three times a week. Over time, increase the time and speed.

Warm up, cool down. Allow 5 minutes or so of stretching and slow movement to allow your body to prepare for exercise. After working out, spend another 5 minutes exercising slowly to cool down.

Listen to your body. Don't exercise through pain. At first, you may feel a little stiff after exercising. But you shouldn't feel pain. If you hurt a joint, or pull a muscle or tendon, stop the activity for several days. Most minor injuries can be healed with RICE—rest, ice, compression, and elevation—and over-the-counter painkillers.

Keep the pace. To condition your heart and lungs, you need to be exercising at a brisk enough pace that you breathe deeply and sweat a bit. However, you still should be able to carry on a conversation.

Watch for warning signs. If you experience any of these symptoms, stop the activity and call your doctor immediately: sudden dizziness, cold sweat, paleness, fainting, and/or pain or pressure in your chest during or after exercising.

Pay attention to the weather. Exercise indoors on a hot day, or outdoors during cooler parts of the day. Wear loose, lightweight clothing and drink lots of water before, during, and after exercising. During colder weather, layer clothing and wear a hat.

Keep with it. Make exercise a priority. Schedule time for it and put it on your calendar. Ask a friend to be an exercise buddy. Join an exercise class. Choose activities you like and that you'll stick with.

Have patience. It'll take time to get into better shape. Fitness experts say a program of moderate activity like brisk walking three times a week will improve the functioning of your heart and blood vessels within 8 to 10 weeks. If you exercise four times weekly, improvement can be seen within 3 to 4 weeks.

Lower Your High Blood Pressure

Nearly one in four Americans has high blood pressure (HBP). Also called hypertension, HBP occurs when small arteries (arterioles) become constricted, which makes it difficult for blood to pass through them. This forces the heart to work harder, straining both the heart and the arteries. As the heart works harder, over time, it can enlarge. If the heart becomes sufficiently enlarged, it may be unable to pump enough blood to the body (a condition called heart failure). Organs denied the blood and oxygen they need can't work properly. HBP can also cause the arteries and arterioles to become scarred and less elastic. This makes them prime candidates for artery-clogging atherosclerosis.

The How-to of Lowering Blood Pressure

Obviously you can't do anything about your gender, family history, age, race, or pre-existing health conditions, all of which can influence your blood pressure. However, you can make these changes to lower your blood pressure:

- Lose excess weight
- Limit alcohol
- Exercise regularly
- Limit your salt intake
- Get enough potassium, calcium, and magnesium
- Stop smoking

We've already talked about losing weight, limiting alcoholic beverages (no more than two drinks per day for men, one for women), and getting enough exercise.

Limit Salt/Get Enough Potassium, Calcium, and Magnesium

If you have HBP, your doctor will likely want you to restrict the salt in your diet. For many people, the amount of table salt (sodium chloride) they eat affects their blood pressure. However, not everyone is "salt sensitive." People who are African American, have hypertension or diabetes, or who are older tend to be more sensitive to dietary salt.

The average American consumes about 4,000 to 6,000 milligrams of salt every day—too much for heart health. Most people should consume no more than 2,400 millgrams of salt a day—about 1 teaspoon.

There are three other minerals you should be concerned about if you have high blood pressure: potassium, calcium, and magnesium. Deficiencies in all three are associated with high blood pressure.

Here are some ideas for reducing dietary sodium and getting enough potassium, calcium, and magnesium:

Keep a salt diary. Write down what you eat and how much sodium each food contains.

Limit processed foods. As much as 75 percent of the salt in American diets comes from processed foods. Opt for fresh, fresh frozen, or canned foods with no added salt.

Check labels. Nutrition labels list the amount of sodium. Watch out for ingredients such as sodium chloride, salt, MSG, and baking powder. Look for labels such as "low sodium," "no salt," "light sodium," "no added salt," etc.

Rinse canned foods. Choose lower-sodium versions of canned products. Rinse the food with fresh water before using.

Don't add salt. Put away the salt shaker and avoid adding salt during cooking.

Shy away from salty snacks. Plenty of foods are obviously loaded with salt—pretzels, chips, salt bagels, pickles, soy sauce, cured foods. Choose lower-salt foods.

Look out for medicines with sodium. Some medicines, especially over-the-counter varieties like antacids, are loaded with sodium.

Eat potassium-rich foods. You need at least 3,500 milligrams of potassium per day, which you can get in a balanced, heart-healthy diet. Include plenty of fresh fruits and vegetables such as peaches, figs, bananas, apricots, lima beans, potatoes, spinach, sweet potatoes, and winter squash. Other foods high in potassium include fish, nuts, low-fat milk products, dried beans and peas, and whole-grain cereals. Caution: If you have kidney disease or high blood potassium, consult your doctor first.

Include sources of calcium. You need at least 1200 milligrams of calcium per day for good health. Include skim or low-fat dairy products (lower-fat varieties have even more calcium than full-fat dairy products). If milk products upset your stomach, try lactose-free dairy products such as lactose-reduced or lactose-free milk.

Eat plenty of magnesium-rich foods. These include whole grains, leafy green vegetables, nuts, seeds, and dried peas and beans. Caution: If you have kidney problems, talk with your doctor first.

Stop Smoking

Quitting smoking is one of the most important things you can do for your heart—and for your overall health. Smoking causes more than 400,000 deaths per year in this country. It's a major cause of CHD and heart attack. Smoking causes as many as 30 percent of the CHD-related deaths in the United States each year. Smoking magnifies other CHD risk factors, multiplying the risk. In fact, if you smoke, you're two to six times more likely to have a heart attack compared with nonsmokers. Smokers who have heart attacks are more likely to die than nonsmokers. Smoking:

- Reduces the ability of the blood to carry oxygen
- Raises "bad" LDL cholesterol
- Decreases "good" HDL cholesterol
- Damages the lining of the coronary arteries, making them more vulnerable to plaque
- Makes the blood coagulate more easily, increasing the risk of blood clots
- May trigger coronary spasm
- May lead to irregular heart rhythms

In addition, cigarette smoking is the biggest risk for *peripheral vascular disease,* narrowing of the blood vessels in the arms and legs. It also increases the risk for several types of cancer, chronic lung diseases, asthma, infertility, and impotence.

Quitting can dramatically lower your risk for heart disease and other health problems, no matter how long you've smoked. The risk to your heart drops soon after you quit. Within two years of quitting smoking, your chances of dying from a heart attack will be cut in half. In ten years, your risk will be nearly the same as for someone who has never smoked (depending on your other risk factors).

People with CHD who've had a heart attack and stop smoking cut their risk of another heart attack, sudden cardiac death, and dying from CHD by 50 percent.

The How-to of Quitting Smoking

Recognize why you want to quit. Before you take the plunge, write down all the reasons you want to quit. Then write down all the benefits you'll receive as a nonsmoker such as saving money, improved health, and cleaner-smelling clothing. Post your list where you'll see it every day. When you're tempted to smoke, review your list.

Talk with your doctor about medical help. You don't have to rely on willpower alone. Your doctor can prescribe nicotine replacement products (patches or gum) to ease your transition to nonsmoking. Nicotine replacements deliver small, steady doses of nicotine without the "buzz" that keeps you hooked. While they contain nicotine, they don't deliver the tar and carbon monoxide responsible for some of the adverse health effects of smoking. An even newer option is the "anti-smoking pill." *Zyban (bupropion hydrochloride)* contains no nicotine but appears to affect chemicals in the brain associated with nicotine addiction. Combined with behavior modification, both nicotine replacement products and Zyban have proven successful for many ex-smokers.

Set a quit date. Mark it on your calendar. Then stick to it.

Get your environment ready. Toss out all cigarettes, ashtrays, lighters, and matches you may have in your home, workplace, or car. Wash your curtains, bedclothes, and anything else that has cigarette smoke odor. Make your environment off-limits to cigarette smoking.

Enlist the support of others. Tell your friends and family you're quitting. Ask them to help.

Recognize and avoid your triggers. Certain situations, people, and places can make you want to smoke. Take some time to list all your triggers. Then avoid them.

Be prepared for withdrawal. Know that you're going to experience some unpleasant sensations when you quit—headache, anxiety, nervousness, cravings, etc. Even people who have smoked for years overcome withdrawal symptoms within two to four weeks. Some people have successfully used acupuncture or hypnosis to combat these symptoms. Others prefer to use temporary nicotine replacement products to lessen withdrawal.

Drink large quantities of water and fruit juices. They will help wash the nicotine out of your body.

Change behaviors. If, for instance, you smoke right after a meal, take a walk instead. If you smoke while driving, carpool with nonsmokers or take the bus.

Exercise. Take up walking, biking, or any other physical activity you enjoy. It'll help you combat the stress of quitting and help your heart and lungs recover.

Learn to relax. Try deep breathing. Take long, deep breaths. Repeat at least five times. Learn to meditate. Listen to relaxation audiotapes or soothing music.

Keep your hands busy. Sew, crochet, carve wood, do crossword puzzles, garden, write letters.

Record and reward your progress. As you reach each new milestone—one week, one month, two months, six months, a year—mark it on the calendar and then do something nice to reward yourself.

Keep a savings bank. In it, put the money you're saving each day from not smoking. Plan to do something wonderful (like take a trip) with the savings.

Don't have "just one." Weeks or months after you quit, don't think you can have "just one" cigarette without getting hooked again.

Get back on the horse. If you smoke after you've quit, don't punish yourself. Just review your reasons for quitting and start again.

10

Alternative Treatments

At this point, you may be saying, "Yes, but aren't there alternatives for me? What about meditation or taking vitamins or herbal supplements? I've heard about alternative ways to clean out the arteries. What about those?" Let's look at what some of the research says about other types of treatment for coronary heart disease.

Stress Management

Do stress and personality traits cause CHD and subsequent heart attacks? This question is still being hotly debated. Much of the research indicates that one's response to stress and the traits of hard-driving personality types (so-called type A's) can increase the risk of heart disease. We don't know if it's how stress influences the body directly or whether it's the unhealthy responses to it (smoking, overeating, drinking, inactivity)—or a combination—that increases CHD risk. Whatever the cause, doctors do know that psychological stress can trigger:

- Increases in blood pressure
- Rapid heart rate
- Narrowing of arteries

- Chest pain
- Activation of clotting agents in the blood
- Release of fats into the bloodstream
- Release of the hormone *cortisol,* which raises blood cholesterol
- Dangerous heart rhythm disturbances (arrhythmias)

What exactly is stress? It's a term used to describe a person's response to physical, emotional, and environmental factors. It's *not* the events or people or situations that frighten, enrage, or annoy us that cause stress. It's our *reaction* to them. All of us know people who just seem to serenely go through life. Things never seem to faze them. Then there are others who react—or overreact—to the least little inconvenience or disap-pointment with anger, hostility, worry, anxiety, depression, and other unhealthy emotions. One study published in *Circulation* found that people who frequently feel depressed are more likely to develop heart disease. Another found the risk of heart attack increases for at least two hours following an angry outburst. Still other studies suggest that a chronic state of stress can cause permanent increases in heart rate, blood pressure, and possibly blood cholesterol, all of which increase the risk of CHD and heart attack.

Most heart experts recommend a program of stress management as a part of an overall treatment plan for CHD. Here are some suggestions to de-stress your life:

Practice Relaxation. A number of techniques are effective in helping people relax and unwind. Take a class to learn to meditate. Do yoga. Buy some progressive relaxation tapes. Ask your doctor for a referral to a qualified practitioner who can teach you biofeedback techniques.

Also, try this deep-breathing exercise. Sit in a quiet, comfortable place where you won't be disturbed. Close your eyes. Take a deep breath in. At the top of your inhalation, hold for 3 to 5 seconds. Then slowly let your breath out, trying to make your exhalation longer than your inhalation. Use your stomach muscles to squeeze out all the air. Then take another deep inhalation, hold, and exhale. Repeat for 5 to 6 breaths.

Exercise Regularly. Aerobic exercise that is rhythmic, uses the large muscles of the arms and legs, and makes you breathe deeply is an excellent stress reducer. Brisk walking, jogging, bicycling, and swimming are all good forms of aerobic exercise. This type of exercise stimulates *endorphins*—the same "feel good" chemicals that runners who experience the "runner's high" talk about.

Get some rest. In this fast-paced world, too many of us are sleep deprived. Not getting enough sleep can leave you fatigued and vulnerable to stress. Most people need at least six to eight hours of sleep a night.

For a good night's sleep:

- Try to go to bed at the same time every night.
- Make your bedroom dark and quiet.
- Avoid caffeinated drinks and foods and exercising late in the day.
- Be careful about the television or radio programs you watch, especially right before going to bed (don't

expect a restful night's sleep after watching stories on national or international crises on the news).

Prioritize. Many people feel stressed because they load up their life with too many things. Learn to prioritize. Look at everything in your life and ask yourself—is this essential? Could someone else do it? Then delegate. Learn to say no to those demands that aren't critical.

Set aside "me" time. Few adults get time all to themselves, yet it's essential for good mental health and for keeping a lid on stress. Give yourself time every day—even if it's only a few minutes—to do something you really enjoy. Go out and pick flowers in your garden. Putter in your shop. Take up a hobby that interests you. Take a class on something you want to learn about.

Develop a support system. People who are socially isolated are at greater risk for serious health problems, including heart disease. Take the time to develop and maintain a group of close, supportive friends. Let your family and friends know you care about them.

Get organized. Nothing stresses like being late or disorganized. Get up 15 minutes earlier or leave a few minutes sooner so that you're not rushing. Set your clothes out the night before. Make an effort to organize areas of your life that are a mess. Perhaps you need a file folder system to organize your bills. Or maybe getting a hook system can help you hang up your keys rather than rushing around frantically looking for them. If you have trouble organizing yourself, there are plenty of organizing professionals who can help.

Volunteer. Nothing helps us get out of ourselves as well as helping someone less fortunate. It can provide a social outlet and possibly a new source of friends as well as the satisfaction of making a worthwhile contribution. Think about things you care about—the environment, older people, the disabled, children's issues, veterans' rights, animals, whatever. Then contact the appropriate organization in your community and ask how you can help.

Vitamins and Other Supplements

Antioxidants

Can you prevent or treat CHD with vitamins or other supplements? It's an attractive thought and one that researchers have been studying. One group of vitamins—the so-called antioxidants—have been attracting a lot of attention for their potential for helping the heart. When cells use oxygen, they produce by-products called free radicals. These free radicals damage cells in a process called *oxidation*. In heart disease, free radicals are believed to be involved in the oxidation of LDL cholesterol, which contributes to atherosclerotic plaque buildup and subsequent heart attacks. Antioxidants can help prevent damage to tissues from oxidation by neutralizing free radicals. Three antioxidants that have received the most attention from researchers are vitamin E, vitamin C, and the carotenoids, such as beta-carotene.

Some studies have shown that high levels of vitamin E are associated with a lower incidence of CHD. In the Cambridge Heart Antioxidant Study (CHAOS), people who took 400 to 800 IUs per day of vitamin E had fewer cardiac events such as heart attacks than those who received a sugar pill (placebo).

However, other studies (such as a recent Canadian study) have found that vitamin E supplements have no effect.

Studies on vitamins A, C, and other antioxidant supplements have been even more disappointing. In fact, people who take statin drugs and niacin and also take vitamin C may lose some of the beneficial effects of the medication, especially related to HDL levels. However, population studies have shown that eating more fruits and vegetables does lower heart disease risk. Research doesn't yet show that supplementing these vitamins in pill form can prevent heart attacks or atherosclerosis. As a result, most heart authorities recommend getting the antioxidants your heart needs from foods rather than pills. Make sure you eat a balanced diet with plenty of antioxidant-rich fruits and vegetables.

Folate/B Vitamins

The amino acid homocysteine is a natural by-product of the body's use of protein and one of the many building blocks of proteins. Recent evidence suggests that elevated levels of homocysteine may be a factor in developing heart disease. Research shows that people who get less than the recommended daily allowance (RDA) of three vitamins—folate (folic acid), vitamin B_6, and vitamin B_{12}—are more likely to have higher levels of homocysteine. (These vitamins help the body process homocysteine.) Elevated homocysteine levels can be lowered by reducing fat in the diet, eating plenty of fresh fruits and vegetables, and getting enough folic acid, vitamin B_6, and vitamin B_{12}. (The RDA for folic acid is 400 micrograms, 2 milligrams for B_6; and 6 micrograms for B_{12}.) It's not been proven that lowering homocysteine levels will prevent heart or blood vessel disease. Studies are still being conducted to see what levels of supplementation are safe and effective for heart disease. In the meantime, eat a balanced diet loaded with fruits and vegetables and take a daily multivitamin that contains the RDA for folic acid, vitamin B_6, and vitamin B_{12}. These three vitamins have been demonstrated to reduce restenosis following angioplasty.

Garlic Supplements

Many people are gulping down garlic supplements in hopes that it will reduce heart disease. Garlic does have some disease-fighting qualities. Animal studies have shown that garlic

Supplements can interfere or interact negatively with some drugs. Talk to your doctor before taking them.

lowers the production of triglycerides and cholesterol in the liver. Evidence shows that garlic thins the blood and makes it less likely that clots will form. It may also help prevent and may even reverse the growth of arterial plaque. However, not everyone is convinced. A recent analysis of several studies found that on average, garlic lowered cholesterol, but that in some of the more rigorous studies garlic performed no better than a placebo.

There are also questions about the form of garlic and dose that's safe and effective. Some authorities suggest that eating garlic as supplements isn't as effective as the natural dietary form because the stomach breaks down the compound largely responsible for the heart-healthy benefits. Cooking garlic may also change the healthy compounds. Eating large amounts of garlic can cause anemia and irritation of the gastrointestinal tract as well as bad breath. Doctors aren't sure what a safe dosage is for supplementation. Because there's little regulation of food supplements, there's also the problem of knowing if what's listed on the label is actually what's in the tablets. For now, eating garlic in your diet is the best way to enjoy it.

Fiber

The indigestible parts of plants, fiber is a proven cancer fighter. It can also lower "bad" LDL cholesterol by 10 to 15 percent. To increase your fiber, eat plenty of fresh fruits and vegetables (including the edible skins), whole grains, beans, and peas. Adding fiber-rich foods such as oat bran to your breakfast is an easy way to increase your fiber intake. The American Heart Association recommends getting 20 to 25 grams of fiber per day for good heart health.

Soy

People in Asian countries have low levels of heart disease and they consume large amounts of soy foods. Natural soy compounds (*isoflavones*) may act like hormones that regulate cholesterol levels. When soy protein is used in place of animal protein, it lowers blood cholesterol levels. Soy's greatest benefit may be that it replaces the intake of other proteins such as meat, which is loaded with cholesterol and saturated fat. Some studies have shown that consuming 25 to 50 grams of soy protein per day is safe and can reduce "bad" LDL cholesterol by up to 8 percent.

Black Tea

Some evidence suggests that black tea may be good for maintaining healthy arteries. A study presented at the American Heart Association's Scientific Sessions 2000 found that the *flavonoids* in black tea improve the function of the inner lining of the arteries. Flavonoids—also found in onions, dark beer, red wine, and red grape juice—help prevent the oxidation of "bad" LDL cholesterol that leads to plaque. The inner lining of the blood vessels is responsible for responding to changes in the body's demands for oxygen and blood by causing the vessels to dilate or narrow. When the lining is healthy, it's also better able to inhibit the formation of blood clots and inflammation of the vessel walls.

Red Wine

If you read newspapers or magazines, you've probably read stories suggesting that drinking red wine may protect against heart disease. The incidence of death from CHD in France, where they consume lots of red wine, is about half that of the United States, despite the fact that the French eat about the same amount of animal fat. Some believe this may be due to the antioxidant properties of flavonoids (also found in dark beer, red grape juice, onions, and black tea) and other compounds such as *resveratrol* in red wine. However, some studies show that it isn't just wine, but any type of distilled spirits that have this heart-protective effect.

Drinking alcohol in moderation (up to one drink a day for women, two for men) appears to lower the risk of heart attack. It also raises the levels of "good" HDL cholesterol and may help prevent blood clots.

Chelation Therapy

Used to treat atherosclerosis since the 1950s, *chelation therapy* involves 30 to 50 intravenous injections of *ethylenediamine tetra-acetic acid* (*EDTA*). The idea is that EDTA binds to minerals in the blood, including calcium, which are then excreted through the urine. Chelation is promoted as sort of a "drain cleaner" for the arteries, softening the plaques by removing the calcium in them. Then the lost minerals are replaced with oral supplements.

Chelation therapy is a proven therapy for removing heavy metals (such as lead) from the blood. However, no scientific studies prove that this expensive alternative therapy works for atherosclerosis. In a recent major randomized placebo controlled study involving 3140 patients published in the *Journal of the American Medical Association*, there was no benefit of chelation. Remember that the calcium measured by EBT (see chapter 6) is simply a *diagnostic marker* for CHD. The real problem with plaque is *not* the calcium, but the cholesterol at the core of the plaque. Medical authorities such as the American Heart Association, the American Medical Association, and the American College of Cardiology do not endorse chelation therapy for treating heart disease. A few years ago, the Food and Drug Administration, charging that chelation therapy has no scientific basis, took steps to prevent its proponents from making claims about its health benefits in treating heart disease.

Work with Your Doctor

Although current research doesn't indicate that most so-called alternative treatments for CHD really help, this doesn't mean that other studies won't find other treatments that are effective in the future. In the meantime, it's important not to be taken in by false claims of unproven treatments or to use such treatments in place of ones that have been scientifically proven to work. Supplements, methods, or procedures that claim to be "secret" cures for heart disease aren't. There aren't secret cures in medicine.

Reputable medical research centers around the world are actively studying treatments for CHD, including many alternative treatments like supplements. Much of the research has resulted in newer, more effective medicines, diagnostic techniques, and treatment procedures like anigioplasty, stenting, and bypass surgery. In the future, CHD treatment will be even more effective. For now, it's important to work closely with your doctor to find the best treatments for you so that you can enjoy a long and healthy life.

Glossary

Alpha-blockers: Blood pressure-lowering drugs that block the stimulation of specialized nerves.

ACE inhibitors (ACEs): Also called angiotensin converting enzyme inhibitors, ACEs belong to a class of drugs used to lower high blood pressure, treat heart failure and patients after heart attacks. ACEs block the formation of the chemical that causes tiny arteries to constrict.

Angina: The medical term is angina pectoris. Angina is chest pressure and pain caused when the heart doesn't receive enough oxygen.

AngioJet: A high-pressure spray device used with a catheter to break up blood clots.

Angioplasty: Also called balloon angioplasty or percutaneous transluminal coronary angioplasty (PTCA), angioplasty is an invasive procedure that treats the inside of coronary arteries without opening the chest.

Angiotensin: A chemical the body produces that causes small arteries (arterioles) to constrict.

Antiarrhythmics: Medications that correct heart rhythm problems.

Anticoagulants: Blood-thinning drugs that inhibit special proteins that form blood clots.

Antiplatelets: Drugs that reduce the ability of the blood to clot by inhibiting the normal function of platelets (blood clotting cells).

Aorta: The large artery that receives blood from the left ventricle and carries it to the body.

Apoproteins: Proteins the body uses to coat cholesterol so that it may be transported in the blood.

Glossary

ARBs: Also called angiotensin receptor blockers, these are drugs prescribed for high blood pressure. They block the chemical that causes tiny arteries to constrict.

Arterioles: Tiny arteries, the blood vessels that carry blood, oxygen, and nutrients to cells in the body.

Arteriosclerosis: Commonly called "hardening of the arteries," arteriosclerosis is a process in which the arteries become thicker and harder, losing their natural elasticity.

Arrhythmia: Abnormal heat-beat.

Artery: A blood vessel that carries blood away from the heart.

Atherosclerosis: A process in which deposits of cholesterol, cellular waste products, calcium, and other substances build up in the inner lining of arteries.

Atriums (or Atria): Top chambers of the heart.

Beta-blockers: A class of drugs often used to alleviate angina and treat high blood pressure. They block adrenaline's effect on the heart, decreasing heart rate, reducing the strength of the heart's contractions, and lowering blood pressure.

Blood pressure: A measurement of the force when the heart pumps blood into the arteries and out to the body and the force of the arteries as they resist the blood from the heart. It's expressed in millimeters of mercury (mmHg).

Brachytherapy: Also called intracoronary radiation, brachytherapy involves exposing the arteries to gamma or beta radiation to reduce the incidence of arterial renarrowing.

Bruits: The rough, turbulent sounds of blood moving through narrowed arteries. Doctors use a stethoscope on the neck, abdomen, and elsewhere to detect bruits (French for noise).

Calcium channel blockers: Drugs that block or inhibit the movement of calcium in the heart, nerves, and blood vessel walls. These drugs reduce blood pressure and dilate coronary arteries.

Capillaries: Very small vessels, often too small to see, that connect the arterial and venous blood systems.

Cardiac angiography: Also called arteriography, angiocardiography, or cardiac catheterization and angiography, this invasive diagnostic technique uses flexible tubes called catheters threaded through the

163

arteries. It can show blood flow problems and blockages in the coronary arteries.

Cardiac positron-emission tomography (PET): An imaging technology that can measure blood flow and metabolism in the heart.

Catheter: A long, slender, flexible tube used in angiography that is threaded through the arteries.

CAT scan: An imaging technique in which an X-ray beam is passed through the body as the scanner is rapidly rotated around the body. It produces a detailed cross section of the body.

Cholesterol: A waxy, fat-like substance that is found in every cell in the body. It is used to help digest fats, strengthen cell membranes, and make some types of hormones and vitamins. It is also a major component of plaque.

Coronary arteries: The arteries that branch from the aorta, divide into smaller arteries, and provide blood for the heart muscle.

Coronary artery bypass graft surgery (CABG): Surgery in which pieces of blood vessels are stitched around blocked arteries, creating bypasses around blockages.

Coronary heart disease (CHD): Also called coronary artery disease (CAD) or ischemic heart disease, it is a condition caused when arteries become narrowed by plaque.

Coronary occlusion: Blockage of a coronary artery that restricts the blood supply.

Coronary thrombosis: Another name for coronary occlusion, a heart attack caused by a clot blocking blood supply to the heart.

Cyanotic: Skin that is bluish in color, which may be a sign of vascular disease or lack of oxygen.

Diabetes: Called diabetes mellitus, it's a disease in which the body isn't able to produce and/or respond to the hormone insulin, which converts blood sugar into energy.

Directional atherectomy: A procedure in which the cardiologist shaves away plaque and removes it from the body.

Dissection of the aorta: A life-threatening condition in which the inner lining of the major artery that leads away from the heart (aorta) becomes torn and may cause severe chest pain.

Diuretics: Drugs that flush excess water and sodium from the body by increasing urination.

Doppler ultrasound: Part of an echocardiogram study that produces heart sounds and displays a picture of the blood flowing between the chambers of the heart.

Echocardiogram: A diagnostic test in which sound waves are used to "bounce back" images of the heart.

Electrocardiography (ECG): A diagnostic test that records the electrical activity of the heart.

Electron beam angiography (EBA): A non-invasive diagnostic technique that produces images of the coronary arteries using injection of X-ray dye using the EBT machine.

Electron beam tomography (EBT): Also called electron beam computed tomography (EBCT), this ultra-fast CT scan detects CHD by measuring calcium in the blood vessels.

Endotracheal tube: A breathing tube used during bypass surgery.

Estrogen: A female hormone. Oral contraceptives and hormone replacement therapy (HRT) use synthetic forms of estrogen.

Exercise ECG: Also called a stress ECG or treadmill test, it's a diagnostic test that records the electrical activity of the heart under stress (exercise or medication).

Fibrates: Triglyceride-lowering medications.

Gene therapy: A new technology for treating disease, gene therapy involves introducing genetic material into cells to cause certain actions.

Heart attack: Also called myocardial infarction, a heart attack occurs when the blood supply to a portion of the heart muscle is blocked and the part of the heart that doesn't receive blood becomes damaged and dies.

Heart failure: A condition in which the heart becomes unable to pump efficiently and supply the body with the blood it needs.

High blood pressure: Also called hypertension, high blood pressure occurs when the blood pressure is 140/90 mm/Hg or higher, which strains the heart.

High-density lipoprotein: So-called good cholesterol, HDL cholesterol contains mostly protein. When there's excess cholesterol in the blood, HDL cholesterol picks up cholesterol deposited in the arteries and transports it to the liver for disposal.

Holter monitoring: Also called ambulatory ECG monitoring, it's a variation of electrocardiography that monitors and records the heart's electrical activity during everyday activities. It's used to detect heart problems that come and go.

Homocysteine: An amino acid that's a by-product of the body's use of protein. High levels of homocysteine have been associated with a low intake of folate, vitamin B_6, and vitamin B_{12} and may be a risk factor for heart disease.

Hydrogenation: A process used in making margarine and shortening in which unsaturated fats become more highly saturated fats.

Instent restenosis: A condition in which arteries that are treated with stents (fine-mesh tubes) become renarrowed.

Insulin: A hormone produced by the pancreas that helps the body convert blood sugar (glucose) into a useable form for energy.

Internal mammary arteries: Two arteries located on the inside chest wall that are often used in bypass surgery.

Intracoronary radiation: Also called brachytherapy, it's a procedure in which arteries treated with stents are exposed to radiation in an effort to stop or slow down the formation of scar tissue.

Intravascular ultrasound (IVUS): An imaging technology in which a small device mounted on the tip of a catheter is inserted into coronary arteries. The device sends back images of the inside of the arteries using ultrasound technology.

Ischemia: Reduced blood flow to an organ. In most cases, this reduction is caused by a blockage or narrowing of an artery.

Ischemic heart disease: Another name for coronary artery disease or coronary heart disease. Ischemic heart disease is caused by arteries that supply the heart becoming narrowed and causing a reduced blood supply to the heart.

Lipoprotein profile: A fasting blood test that measures total cholesterol, HDL and LDL cholesterol, and triglyceride levels. All adults should have a lipoprotein profile performed at least once every five years.

Lipoproteins: The protein "packages" that transport cholesterol in the blood.

Low-density lipoprotein: So-called bad cholesterol, LDL cholesterol contributes to plaque building in the arteries.

Magnetic Resonance Imaging (MRI): Formerly called nuclear magnetic resonance (NMR), this diagnostic test uses powerful magnets and radio waves to produce images of the inside of the body.

Myocardial infarction (MI): The medical term for heart attack. When blood supply to a part of the heart is severely reduced or blocked, a heart attack can occur. The area of the heart muscle on the other side of the blockage begins to die and results in permanent damage to the heart.

Nicotinic acid: The B vitamin niacin that's used to decrease LDL cholesterol and triglycerides and increase HDL cholesterol.

Nitrate: A type of anti-anginal medication used to widen the coronary arteries.

Nuclear scanning: A variety of diagnostic tests that involve injecting a tiny amount of radioactive material into the bloodstream and taking images of the radiation given off by the material.

Pericarditis: Inflammation of the fibrous sac that surrounds the heart (pericardium). The chest pain caused by pericarditis can mimic angina.

Plaque: A mixture of fatty substances, cholesterol, cellular waste products, calcium, and other substances that become deposited in the inner lining of arteries.

Platelets: The clotting cells in blood.

Pressure wire: A diagnostic tool used in the cath lab that measures pressures inside arteries to determine the significance of a narrowing.

Progestin: A synthetic form of the female hormone progesterone. Progestin is often used in birth control pills and hormone replacement therapy (HRT).

Pulmonary embolism: Blood clot in the lung.

Pump oxygenator: Commonly called a heart-lung machine, it's used to keep the blood flowing and oxygenated while the heart is stopped during surgery.

Reperfusion therapy: A variety of techniques (including medications, angioplasty, and surgery) that may be used to restore blood flow to areas of the heart damaged by a heart attack.

Resins: Cholesterol-lowering drugs that cause the intestines to absorb less cholesterol from the digestive tract.

Restenosis: The term used when arteries become narrowed again following a procedure to open them.

Risk factors: Traits or lifestyle habits that put one at greater risk for developing certain illnesses or conditions.

Rotational atherectomy: A procedure in which the cardiologist uses a diamond-coated burr to treat conditions such as calcified plaque.

Saphenous vein: The vein that lies just inside the leg. It's often used in bypass surgery.

Saturated fat: The type of fat that comes from animal sources (meat, poultry, egg yolks, dairy products). Solid at room temperature, saturated fat has been associated with the plaque building of atherosclerosis.

Silent ischemia: A temporary shortage of blood and oxygen to the heart that doesn't produce any symptoms.

Single photon emission computed tomography (SPECT): One of the most commonly used nuclear imaging technologies. It involves injecting a radioactive material and then taking images of the chest.

Statins: Drugs often used to reduce cholesterol, statins work directly on the liver to block the manufacture of cholesterol.

Stenosis: Narrowing. In the case of CHD, narrowing of blood vessels.

Stents: Small, fine-mesh tubes that are inserted into arteries to keep them open.

Stroke: Also called a "brain attack," a stroke occurs when one or more blood vessels supplying the brain become blocked, causing the death of brain cells.

Sudden cardiac death (SCD): Sudden and unexpected death caused by the total loss of heart function in someone with or without diagnosed heart disease.

Tachycardia: Abnormally rapid heartbeat.

Thrombolytics: Clot-busting drugs used in the treatment of heart attack.

Total blood cholesterol: A combination of low-density lipoprotein (LDL) and high-density lipoprotein (HDL) cholesterol and triglycerides.

Transmyocardial revascularization (TMR): A technique in which the surgeon drills laser holes into the heart's pumping chamber to relieve chest pain.

Triglycerides: A type of blood fat. Elevated levels of triglycerides are associated with CHD.

Glossary

Variant angina: Also called Prinzmetal's angina, it's a less common type of chest pain caused when the muscle fibers surrounding the coronary arteries spasm and narrow or completely close off blood vessels that feed the heart.

Vasodilators: Medications that reduce blood pressure by dilating blood vessels.

Vein: One of many vessels that carry blood to the heart.

Ventricles: The lower chambers of the heart (one right and one left).

Venules: Small veins.

Very-low-density lipoprotein (VLDL): A type of cholesterol-protein package that contains cholesterol, triglycerides, and protein.

Resources

American Heart Association

National Center
7272 Grandville Avenue
Dallas, TX 75231
800-AHA-USA1 (242-8721)
www.americanheart.org

The American Heart Association's mission is to reduce disability and death from cardiovascular diseases and stroke. It is a not-for-profit, voluntary health organization funded by private contributions. The web site offers links to message boards, chat rooms, patient guides, caregiver guides, and nutrition and recipe information. The site also features an "Ask the Expert" section.

National Heart, Lung, and Blood Institute (NHLBI)

P.O. Box 30105
Bethesda, MD 20824
301-251-1222
www.nhlbi.nih.gov

The National Heart, Lung, and Blood Institute (NHLBI) provides leadership for a national program in diseases of the heart, blood vessels, lung, and blood; blood resources; and sleep disorders. The Institute plans, conducts, fosters, and supports an integrated and coordinated program of basic research, clinical investigations and trials, observational studies, and demonstration and education projects.

National Institute of Neurological Disorders and Stroke (NINDS)

P.O. Box 5801
Bethesda, MD 20824
800-352-9424
www.ninds.nih.gov

Serving the public and health professionals, the organization offers comprehensive consumer health information, publications, new treatment studies, clinical studies, clinical research training and research funding.

Pulmonary Hypertension Association

P.O. Box 463,
Ambler, PA 19002
Phone: 800-748-7274
www.phassociation.org

Support and information for patients with pulmonary hypertension, their families and physicians. Encourages research, promotes awareness, provides resource references. Networking, phone help, pen pals, assistance in starting groups.

Adult Congenital Heart Association (ACHA)

273 Perham Street
West Roxbury, MA 02132
www.achaheart.org

The Adult Congenital Heart Association (ACHA) is a national organization for adults and adolescents with congenital heart disease (CHD). The purpose of our organization is to educate the public, adults with CHD, and the medical community about adult congenital heart issues through the development of forums, newsletters, support groups, and message boards.

American Society of Nuclear Cardiology (ASNC)

9111 Old Georgetown Road
Bethesda, MD 20814
301-493-2360
www.asnc.org

The American Society of Nuclear Cardiology (ASNC) is a professional medical society. The mission of ASNC is to foster optimal delivery of

Nuclear Cardiology services through developing standards of
professional education and training, establishing guidelines for the
clinical performance of Nuclear Cardiology, and the promotion of
Nuclear Cardiology research.

Heart Failure Society of America, Inc.

Court International–Suite 238N
2550 University Avenue West
Saint Paul, Minnesota 55114
651-642-1633
www.hfsa.org

The Heart Failure Society of America, Inc. (HFSA) represents the efforts
by heart failure experts from the Americas to provide a forum for all
those interested in heart function, heart failure, and congestive heart
failure (CHF) research and patient care.

The Mended Hearts, Inc.

7272 Greenville Avenue
Dallas, Texas 75231-4596
214-706-1442
www.mendedhearts.org

A nationwide patient support organization is comprised of people with
heart disease, their families, medical professionals, and other interested
persons.

The Coronary Club, Inc.

9500 Euclid Avenue
Mail Code A42
Cleveland, OH 44195
800-478-4255

The Coronary Club, a nonprofit organization, was founded in 1968 to
provide patients and their families with information on preventing heart
attacks and adjusting to life with a heart condition. Subscribers receive
up-to-date reports on coronary care and treatment, diet and exercise,
stress management, surgery, and medications. Local chapters hold
meetings, where members can exchange experiences and hear
speakers.

American Academy of Family Physicians Foundation
11400 Tomahawk Creek Parkway
Leawood, KS 66211-2672
www.familydoctor.org

This organization offers consumer-friendly advise from their book, *Family Health and Medical Guide.*

All of the information has been written and reviewed by physicians and patient education professionals at the American Academy of Family Physicians. The information is regularly reviewed and updated.

The American Alliance for Health, Physical Education, Recreation & Dance
1900 Association Dr.
Reston, VA 20192-1598
1-800-213-7193
www.aahperd.org

AAHPERD is an alliance of six national associations, six district associations, and a research consortium all designed to provide members with a comprehensive resources , support, and programs to help practitioners improve their skills and so further the health and well-being of the American public.

MEDLINE
www.nih.gov

Produced by the National Library of Medicine, this web site indexes articles from more than 3,500 medical journals. The service is aimed primarily at scientists and health professionals. MEDLINEPlus is the lay public's version and is found at: www.nlm.nih.gov/medlineplus.

NOAH New York Online Access to Health
www.noah-health.org

A consortium of library and medical organizations (the City University of New York, the Metropolitan New York Library Council, the New York Academy of Medicine, and the New York Public Library) have combined efforts to give consumers free access to many of the best consumer-oriented health materials by respected sources.

Index

About the Authors

Barry **M. Cohen**, M.D,. F.A.C.C., F.S.C.A.I., is a senior interventional cardiologist at Morristown Memorial Hospital in Morristown, New Jersey. A leader in interventional cardiology research, Dr. Cohen is a graduate of McGill University and the Medical School at the University of Sherbrooke in Sherbrooke, Quebec, Canada. Dr. Cohen did his cardiology fellowship at the MSMC in New York and was a post-doctoral scholar at the University of California-San Diego in interventional cardiology.

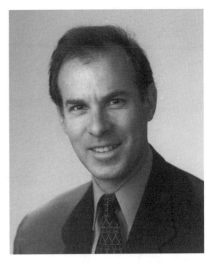

Dr. Cohen is the principal investigator of numerous studies on the treatment of coronary heart disease (CHD). He has investigated new stent designs, arterial protective devices, and refinements in rotational atherectomy techniques. He was involved in the development of an intracoronary brachytherapy program and is investigating the use of gene therapy for patients with CHD and severe angina. Dr. Cohen was the first to perform rotational atherectomy in the New York-New Jersey region, and he has taught this technique in the United States and abroad. He is a leader in computerized cardiac mapping with the Biosense NOGA™ system. Dr. Cohen is a past president of the New Jersey Society of Interventional Cardiology, and is board-certified in internal medicine, cardiovascular disease, and interventional cardiology.

Bobbie Hasselbring is an award-winning health writer who has authored or co-authored more than a dozen books on health and psychology. Ms. Hasselbring was a senior editor for *Medical Self-Care*, a national consumer health magazine. She has written for national and regional newspapers and magazines, and the World Wide Web. She has produced materials for multinational health corporations, pharmaceutical companies, medical publishers, and medical institutions. Ms. Hasselbring has been recognized twice by the American Heart Association for her writing about heart disease and recently won the Rx Club's Excellence in Writing award.

Addicus Books
www.AddicusBooks.com

Please send

_____ copies of _____ at _____ each _____

Shipping & handling $4.00 _____

$1.10 for each additional copy _____

Total: _____

Name_____

Address_____

City _____ State ____ Zip _____

Phone ( ) _____

☐ Visa ☐ MasterCard ☐ American Express

Credit Card Number _____ Exp. Date _____

Order by credit card, personal check or money order. Send to:

Addicus Books
Mail Order Dept.
P.O. Box 45327
Omaha, NE 68145
Or, order **TOLL FREE: 800-352-2873**